ORAL COMPLICATIONS OF CANCER CHEMOTHERAPY

Previously published in this series:

F.J. Cleton and J.W.I.M. Simons, eds., Genetic Origins of Tumor Cells
ISBN 90-247-2272-1

J. Aisner and P. Chang, eds., Cancer Treatment Research
ISBN 90-247-2358-2

B.W. Ongerboer de Visser, D.A. Bosch and W.M.H. van Woerkom-Eykenboom, eds., Neuro-Oncology: Clinical and Experimental Aspects
ISBN 90-247-2421-X

K. Hellmann, P. Hilgard and S. Eccles, eds., Metastasis: Clinical and Experimental Aspects
ISBN 90-247-2424-4

H.F. Seigler, ed., Clinical Management of Melanoma
ISBN 90-247-2584-4

P. Correa and W. Haenszel, eds., Epidemiology of Cancer of the Digestive Tract
ISBN 90-247-2601-8

L.A. Liotta and I.R. Hart, eds., Tumor Invasion and Metastasis
ISBN 90-247-2611-5

J. Bánóczy, ed., Oral Leukoplakia
ISBN 90-247-2655-7

C. Tijssen, M. Halprin and L. Endtz, eds., Familial Brain Tumours
ISBN 90-247-2691-3

E.M. Muggia, C.W. Young and S.K. Carter, eds., Anthracycline Antibiotics in Cancer
ISBN 90-247-2711-1

B.W. Hancock, ed., Assessment of Tumour Response
ISBN 90-247-2712-X

ORAL COMPLICATIONS OF CANCER CHEMOTHERAPY

edited by

DOUGLAS E. PETERSON
Baltimore College of Dental Surgery
Department of Oral Diagnosis
and the University of Maryland School of Medicine
Baltimore, MD, USA

STEPHEN T. SONIS
Division of Dentistry
Brigham and Women's Hospital
and the Harvard School of Dental Medicine
Boston, MA, USA

MARTINUS NIJHOFF PUBLISHERS
The Hague/Boston/London

Distributors:

for the United States and Canada

Kluwer Boston, Inc.
190 Old Derby Street
Hingham, MA 02043

for all other Countries

Kluwer Academic Publishers Group
Distribution Center
P.O. Box 322
3300 AH Dordrecht
The Netherlands

Library of Congress Cataloging in Publication Data

Main entry under title:

Oral complications of cancer chemotherapy.

(Developments in oncology; 12)
Includes bibliographical references and index.
1. Mouth—Diseases. 2. Cancer—Chemotherapy—Complications and sequelae. 3. Antineoplastic agents—Side effects. I. Peterson, Douglas E. II. Sonis, Stephen T. III. Series. [DNLM: 1. Antineoplastic agents—Adverse effects. 2. Mouth diseases—Etiology.
W1 DE998N v. 12 / QZ 267 063]
RC815.067 1983 617′.522 82-22326
ISBN-13: 978-1-4613-3914-4 e-ISBN-13: 978-1-4613-3912-0
DOI: 10.1007/978-1-4613-3912-0

CONTENTS

CONTRIBUTING AUTHORS

Joseph Aisner, M.D.
Head, Division of Medical Oncology
Deputy Director for Clinical Affairs
University of Maryland Cancer Center
University of Maryland Hospital

Associate Professor of Medicine
University of Maryland School of Medicine
Baltimore, MD 21201

Nicholas R. Bachur, M.D., Ph.D.
Chief, Laboratory of Clinical Biochemistry
Baltimore Cancer Research Program
Division of Cancer Treatment
National Cancer Institute
National Institutes of Health
Baltimore, MD 21201

Lee R. Brown, Ph.D.
Professor of Pathology (Microbiology)
University of Texas Dental Branch

Professor
University of Texas Dental Science Institute
Houston, TX 77025

Samuel Dreizen, D.D.S., M.D.
Professor and Chairman
Department of Dental Oncology
University of Texas Dental Branch

Professor
University of Texas Dental Science Institute
Houston, TX 77025

Kenneth T. Izutsu, Ph.D.
Research Associate Professor
Department of Oral Medicine
Department of Oral Biology
University of Washington School of Dentistry
Seattle, WA 98195

Peter B. Lockhart, D.D.S.
Program Director
General Practice Residency Program
Brigham and Women's Hospital

Associate Physician
Sidney Farber Cancer Institute

Assistant Professor
Department of Oral Medicine and Oral Pathology
Harvard School of Dental Medicine
Boston, MA 02115

Joyce L. O'Dwyer R.N., B.S.N.
Patient Education Coordinator
University of Maryland Cancer Center
University of Maryland Hospital
Baltimore, MD 21201

C. Daniel Overholser, D.D.S., M.S.
Associate Professor and Chairman
Department of Oral Diagnosis
Baltimore College of Dental Surgery
Dental School

Assistant Professor
Oncology
University of Maryland School of Medicine
University of Maryland at Baltimore
Baltimore, MD 21201

Douglas E. Peterson, D.M.D., Ph.D.
Associate Professor
Department of Oral Diagnosis
Baltimore College of Dental Surgery
Dental School

Assistant Professor
Oncology
University of Maryland School of Medicine
University of Maryland at Baltimore
Baltimore, MD 21201

Stephen C. Schimpff, M.D.
Director
University of Maryland Cancer Center
University of Maryland Hospital

Professor of Medicine
University of Maryland School of Medicine
Baltimore, MD 21201

Mark M. Schubert, D.D.S., M.S.D.
Lecturer
Department of Oral Medicine
University of Washington School of Dentistry
Seattle, WA 98195

Director, Oral Medicine Support Services
Fred Hutchinson Cancer Research Center
Seattle, WA 98124

Stephen T. Sonis, D.M.D., D.M.Sc.
Chief, Division of Dentistry
Brigham and Women's Hospital

Associate Physician
Sidney Farber Cancer Institute

Associate Professor
Department of Oral Medicine and Oral Pathology
Harvard School of Dental Medicine
Boston, MA 02115

Keith M. Sullivan, M.D.
Assistant Professor of Medicine
University of Washington School of Medicine
Seattle, WA 98195

Assistant Member
Fred Hutchinson Cancer Research Center
Seattle, WA 98124

Edmond L. Truelove, D.D.S., M.S.D.
Associate Professor and Chairman
Department of Oral Medicine
University of Washington School of Dentistry
Seattle, WA 98195

Lisa T. Williams, B.S., R.D.H.
Dental Hygienist
University of Maryland Cancer Center
University of Maryland Hospital

Instructor
Department of Oral Diagnosis
Baltimore College of Dental Surgery
Dental School
University of Maryland at Baltimore
Baltimore, MD 21201

FOREWORD

This new work on oral complications of cancer chemotherapy is edited by two dentists who have made pioneering contributions in this previously neglected area. Their efforts have established the invaluable role of the dentist in oncologic research and cancer patient management.

The editors have collected nine chapters that will be of interest to dentists and dental hygienists, oncology nurses, and all physicians treating cancer patients with chemotherapeutic agents.

Background chapters on oral complications of cancer chemotherapy, the pharmacology of chemotherapeutic agents, and principles of infection management and prevention set the stage for more specific chapters focusing on prevention and treatment of chemotherapy-induced oral and dental disorders.

Valuable contributions to the supportive care of the cancer patient are contained in this book. A full comprehension of this book, coupled with an appreciation for advances in other areas of supportive care, such as antiemetic therapy and pain control, will allow all those involved in cancer treatment to be more successful.

Peter H. Wiernik, M.D.
Emil Frei, M.D.

PREFACE

Results of a number of studies demonstrate that the successful management of the patient with malignant disease is a function not only of direct cancericidal therapy but of aggressive supportive care as well. As the use of chemotherapy has expanded, complications secondary to such treatment have also increased to a point where they may reduce the quality and duration of survival of the patient. Although advances in cancer treatment have been impressive, oral morbidity associated with the disease and its treatment remains a significant problem. Oral pain and ulceration, systemic infectious complications, and nutritional impairment can be common sequelae in myelosuppressed cancer patients.

At the present time, a number of disciplines routinely deal with the diagnosis and management of these and other oral complications of chemotherapy. While large cancer centers may have access to comprehensive dental services, at other institutions the medical oncologist or oncology nurse may have total responsibility for oral care. This book is designed to present, from a broadly based perspective, the current understanding of oral complications that occur secondary to cancer chemotherapy. Included are discussions defining the epidemiology and mechanisms of oral complications and their relationship to systemic infection. The book is pragmatic in that specific management recommendations are discussed in a number of chapters. Where possible, we have attempted to maximize use of published studies; however, on occasion, we have included time-honored, empirically based recommendations. Resource management as it relates to the evaluation, prevention, and treatment of oral complications is the subject of a separate chapter. We feel that the entire health team involved in the management of patients who receive chemotherapy will find this text a useful adjunct in the supportive care of these patients.

ORAL COMPLICATIONS OF CANCER CHEMOTHERAPY

1. EPIDEMIOLOGY, FREQUENCY, DISTRIBUTION, MECHANISMS, AND HISTOPATHOLOGY

STEPHEN T. SONIS, D.M.D., D.M.Sc.

INTRODUCTION

The number of newly diagnosed patients with malignant disease continues to rise annually. Fortunately, the prognostic outlook for these individuals is no longer universally grim. Significant progress has been made in understanding cancer biology and natural defense mechanisms and in the development of new and aggressive treatment modalities. There is evidence of an overall increase in survival time and, in a growing number of cases, the opportunity for curative therapy.

Destruction of malignant cells by tumoricidal chemotherapeutic drugs has proven to be an effective treatment for a variety of malignancies. Like radiotherapy, the antitumor effect of cancer chemotherapeutic agents is based on their ability to nonspecifically destroy or retard the division of rapidly proliferating cells, such as tumor cells. Unfortunately, nonmalignant cells that have a high mitotic index are present in a variety of body compartments, including the gastrointestinal tract and bone marrow, and are subject to the toxic effect of cancer chemotherapy. The oral mucosa with its rapid cell turnover and frequent trauma is a major site of toxicity [1,2]. In addition, the oral cavity's diffuse bacterial flora and the almost ubiquitous presence of chronic infection highlight the mouth's importance as a potential portal of entry for infectious agents in the myelosuppressed cancer patient [3,4].

At present, approximately 20% of patients with cancer are treated with chemotherapy at some phase during their disease. Of patients with malignancies, other than of the head and neck, 40% develop oral complications associated with their therapy [1]. Obviously, this number is greater for patients being treated for head and neck cancers. In absolute

D.E. Peterson and S.T. Sonis (eds.), ORAL COMPLICATIONS OF CANCER CHEMOTHERAPY, 1-12.

numbers, of approximately 785,000 newly diagnosed cancer patients, over 60,000 will have problems associated with their mouths. If one also includes patients who are not newly diagnosed, but are in the midst of ongoing treatment (estimated at about 750,000), another 60,000 patients can be added to the total who can expect to develop oral complications associated with their therapy. It is likely that the number of episodes of oral complications of cancer chemotherapy is even higher than the preceding numbers suggest, since the administration of multiple courses of multiple drugs frequently produces recurrent oral complications in the same individual. Thus one can estimate that there will be approximately 250,000 episodes of oral complications associated with the use of cancer chemotherapy in the United States this year. Clearly, this represents a significant problem to the patient and the therapist since pain, dysfunction, weight loss, bleeding, and infection can arise.

It seems probable that both the number and severity of cancer chemotherapy-induced oral complications will increase. New, more potent drugs, higher doses of drugs, multimodality therapy combining radiation with chemotherapy, multidrug therapy, and an increased ability to manage prolonged myelosuppression all add to the likelihood that the frequency of oral complications will increase.

MECHANISM OF ACTION

Although a variety of oral problems occur as a consequence of cancer chemotherapy (table 1–1), they are fundamentally a consequence of either the direct effect of drugs on the oral mucosa or of an indirect result of myelosuppression (figure 1–1).

Direct stomatotoxicity

Direct stomatotoxicity is caused by the cytotoxic action of chemotherapeutic agents on oral mucosal cells. A decrease in renewal rate of the basal epithelium results in atrophic thinning of the oral mucosa [5]. Clinically, patients experience discomfort; the oral mucosa becomes erythematous and ulcerative. Ulcerations usually begin as discreet lesions and progress to become diffuse and confluent. Direct stomatotoxicity most commonly occurs on the nonkeratinized mucosal surfaces of the mouth such as the buccal and labial mucosa, ventral surface and sides of the tongue, the soft palate and the floor of the mouth, but is rare on the attached gingiva and hard palate. Breakdown of the mucosa is sharply demarcated from unaffected skin at the mucocutaneous junction of the lips (figure 1–2). Since these changes are due to the direct effects of the drug, this form of stomatotoxicity is usually observed within one week (four to seven days) following the administration of the chemotherapeutic agent [6]. Chemotherapeutic agents which routinely produce direct stomatotoxicity include

Table 1–1. Description and frequency of oral complications in 177 patients treated with cancer chemotherapy

Complication	Frequency
Ulceration and mucositis	32%
Xerostomia	16%
Infection (all types)	26%
Gingival breakdown (local)	8%
Oral pain	7%
Hemorrhage	3%

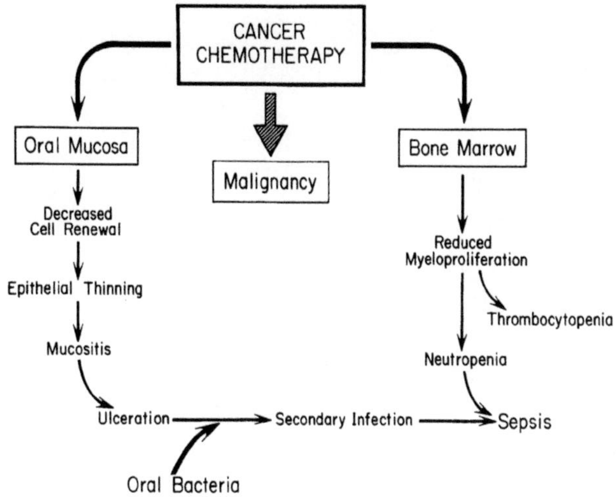

Figure 1–1. Mechanisms responsible for oral complications of cancer chemotherapy. The tumoricidal agent nonspecifically affects dividing cells in the oral basal epithelium and in the bone marrow. Mucosal atrophy and ulceration (direct stomatotoxicity) and infection and bleeding secondary to myelosuppression (indirect stomatotoxicity) may occur.

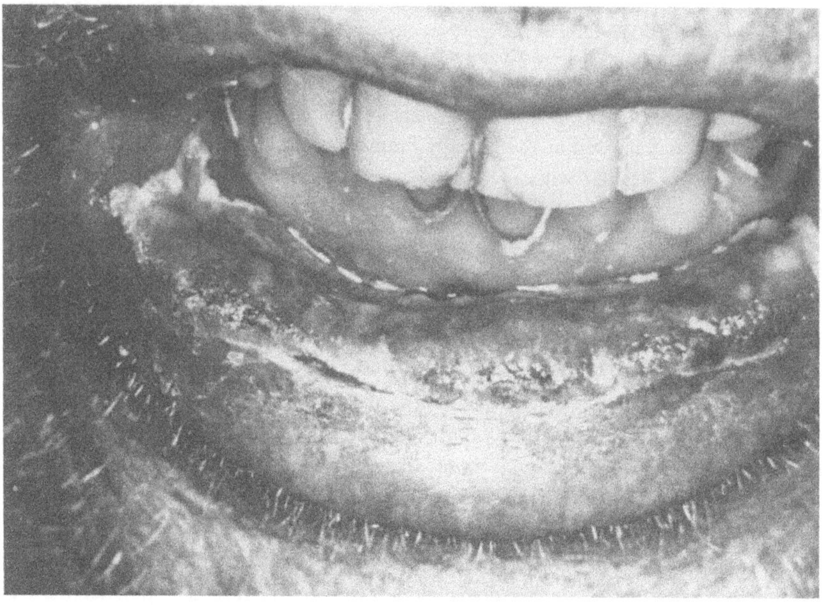

Figure 1–2. Direct stomatotoxicity secondary to methotrexate administration in a 55-year-old male being treated for diffuse histiocytic lymphoma. Note the extent of ulceration on the mandibular labial mucosa, the sharp demarcation between the mucosa and the mucocutaneous junction, and the lack of involvement of the gingiva.

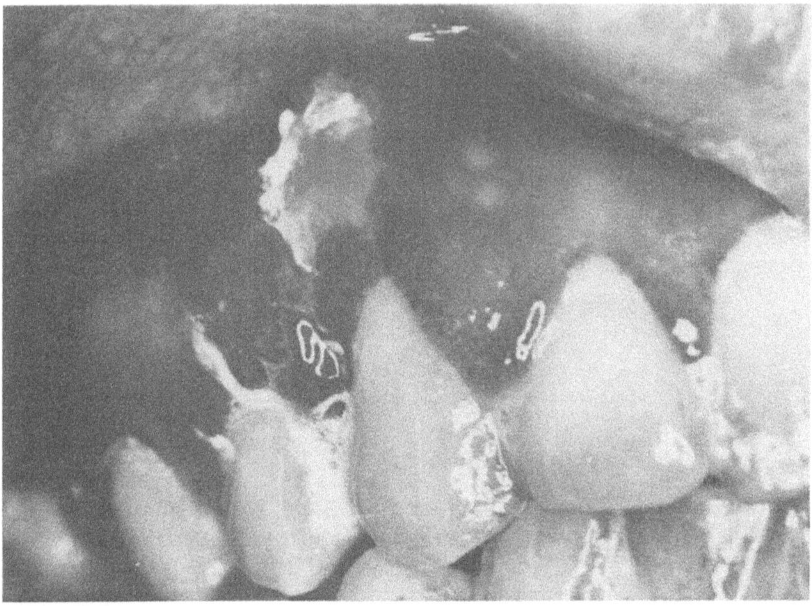

Figure 1–3. Gingival necrosis and secondary infection in a 30-year-old female being treated for acute myelogenous leukemia. This form of indirect stomatotoxicity frequently occurs in patients with preexisting periodontal disease and is generally accompanied by pain and fever.

methotrexate, Adriamycin, 5-fluorouracil, bleomycin, and cytosine arabinoside. Effects of direct stomatotoxicity, although clinically dramatic and painful, are usually self-limiting, with spontaneous healing without scarring occurring about two to three weeks from the time the drug was given.

Indirect stomatotoxicity

Indirect stomatotoxicity is the result of the effects of the chemotherapeutic agent on a cell pool other than that of the oral mucosa. The most significant target cells in this case are those of the bone marrow. Myelosuppression, as manifested by leukopenia and neutropenia, thrombocytopenia, and anemia, is a common sequela of many forms of cancer chemotherapy. Changes in the oral cavity are usually observed 12 to 16 days following the administration of the drug at the nadir of white blood count when the patient is profoundly neutropenic [6,7]. Any agent that causes myelosuppression may produce indirect stomatotoxicity.

Clinically, the effects of neutropenia are initially and most frequently noted in areas of the marginal, papillary and attached gingiva where preexisting chronic infection may predispose the patient to further destruction and infection (chapter 5). Once the initial breakdown of the gingiva is established, ulcerative lesions with surface necrosis may spread to any area of the mucosa (figure 1–3). Secondary infection and bleeding are common. However, the cardinal signs of inflammation are often significantly reduced or absent because of the patient's marrow status.

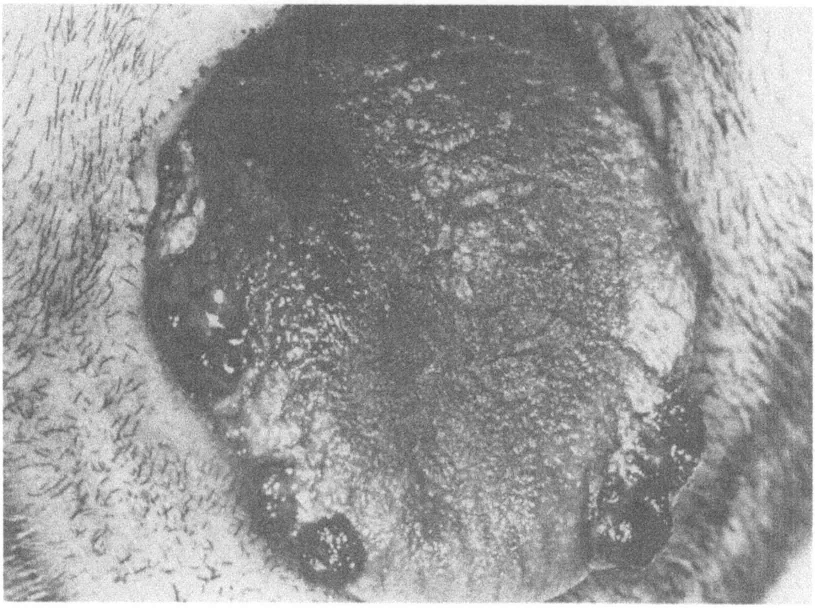

Figure 1–4. Multiple hematomas on the lateral borders of the tongue in a 42-year-old male with thrombocytopenia secondary to chemotherapy (indirect stomatotoxicity).

Hemorrhage is a common sequela of myelosuppression and the resultant thrombocytopenia. Although oral bleeding is frequently an accurate clinical index of thrombocytopenia [8,9], much individual variation is noted among patients. Moreover, greater than 57% of patients with oral bleeding have platelet counts under 60,000 cells/mm^3. Spontaneous gingival bleeding occurs with platelet counts of approximately 15,000 to 20,000 cells/mm^3 [8]. As with other forms of indirect stomatotoxicity, patients with underlying periodontal disease are more likely to develop hemorrhage than are patients with good gingival health. Hematoma formation may occur at any point in the mucosa but is especially common in those areas that are frequently traumatized such as the lateral borders of the tongue (figure 1–4) and the buccal mucosa. Organization of the hematoma is followed by the formation of a fibrin plug (figure 1–5). Before epithelialization is complete, these areas may act as sources of secondary infection and must be followed closely (chapter 7). Hematoma formation of the floor of the mouth is especially worrisome in that profound bleeding may ultimately produce displacement of the tongue and then respiratory embarrassment.

Neurotoxicity is a fairly rare form of indirect stomatotoxicity which occurs most often following the administration of the plant alkaloid, vincristine [1]. Clinically, patients complain of intermittent odontogenic-like pain in one or more mandibular teeth. Radiographic widening of the periodontal ligament space may be noted. The effect is transient and does not represent pulpal degeneration.

Recovery from indirect stomatotoxicity is usually complete by 21 to 24 days following the initiation of chemotherapy [6].

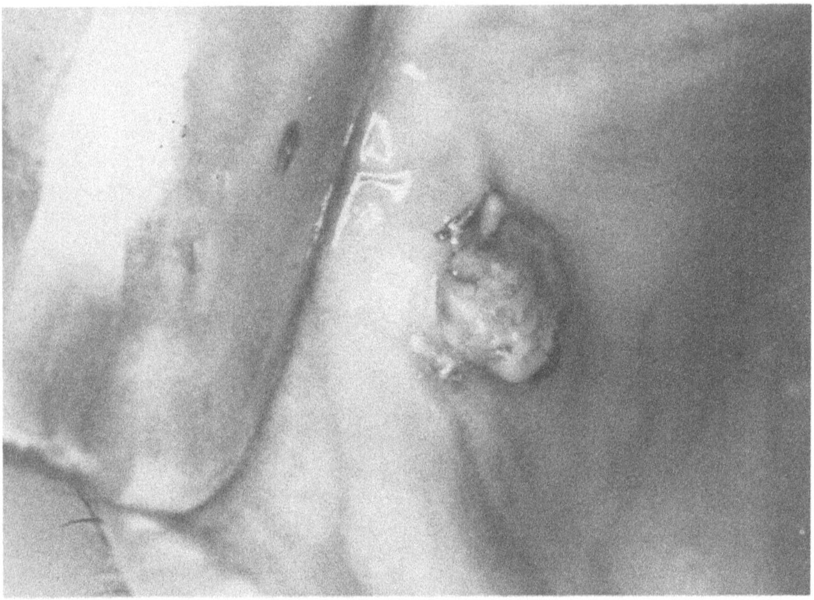

Figure 1–5. Resolving hematoma (fibrin plug) of labial mucosa in a 40-year-old female being treated for acute myelogenous leukemia. The organizing clot offers a potential site for secondary infection in the neutropenic patient. Healing occurs by epithelialization beneath the fibrin plug.

FACTORS THAT INFLUENCE THE FREQUENCY AND SEVERITY OF COMPLICATIONS

The factors that influence the frequency and severity of oral complications of cancer chemotherapy may be broadly divided into two major groups: those that are patient-related and those that are therapy-related (table 1–2). Among the patient-related factors are type of malignancy, patient age, prechemotherapy condition of the mouth, and the level of oral care during chemotherapy. Therapy-related variables include those that are related to the specific drug used for chemotherapy, the total dose of the drug, the timing of delivery of the chemotherapy, and concommitant therapy given with chemotherapy.

Table 1–2. Patient- and therapy-related variables that affect the frequency and severity of oral complications of cancer chemotherapy

Patient-Related	Therapy-Related
Type of malignancy	Drug
Patient age	Total dose
Pretreatment condition of mouth	Drug schedule
Level of oral care during treatment	Concommitant therapy

Patient-related variables

Patients receiving chemotherapy for hematologic malignancies tend to incur oral complications at a higher rate than other forms of malignancy (table 1–3) [1,2]. For example, more than two-thirds of patients with leukemia (especially acute leukemia) can be expected to develop oral complications at some point during the course of their treatment [1]. One-third of patients with non-Hodgkin's lymphomas will develop oral complications [1]. It seems likely that the patient's preexisting compromised hematologic function accentuates the myelosuppressive effects of chemotherapy as well as reduces local oral resistance to infection. The finding of malignant cells of gingival sulcus origin in the saliva of patients with acute lymphocytic leukemia documents their presence in the oral environment and may explain, in part, the susceptibility of these patients to infection of the gingiva and related structures [10]. Patients receiving therapy for solid tumors are at less risk to develop complications of chemotherapy, although these problems do occur at a relatively frequent rate in patients with malignancies of the gastrointestinal tract [20%] and those with carcinoma of the breast [12%]. In the case of solid tumors, almost all oral complications are due to direct stomatotoxicity.

Interestingly, patient age may be a predisposing factor to the development of oral complications of chemotherapy. Both the severity of such complications and length of time that they are present may also be influenced by the patient's age (table 1–4). It appears that the younger the patient, the more likely it is that chemotherapy-induced oral complications will develop [1,2]. Clearly, this observation is, in part, attributable to the fact that leukemia is the most common form of malignancy in young patients and, as already noted, patients with this diagnosis are at increased risk to develop oral problems. However, when patients of different ages with identical malignancies and therapy are compared, this observation remains. Barakat and co-workers have reported that regeneration of the oral mucosa slows with age [11]. In addition, the mitotic index of the mucosa of young individuals may be

Table 1–3. Frequency of oral complications as a function of type of malignancy

Disease	% of Patients with Oral Complications of Patients with Diagnosis
Leukemia (all types)	68%
Non-Hodgkin's lymphomas	33%
Malignancy of gastrointestinal tract	20%
Malignancy of breast	12%

Table 1–4. Frequency of oral complications as a function of patient age

Age Group	Frequency of Oral Complications (%)
1 to 20	90
21 to 40	60
41 to 60	28
> 61	18

greater than in older patients. This latter observation may account for the clinical finding that although younger patients develop severe ulcerations and mucositis secondary to many forms of chemotherapy, they tend to make more rapid and complete recoveries following the cessation of drug than older patients [2].

The condition of the patient's mouth before chemotherapy seems to be significant in determining the frequency and severity of oral complications. Patients with preexisting oral disease, such as periodontal disease or pulpal disease, have an increased frequency of problems following the administration of chemotherapy. Work by Overholser [12] and others which has demonstrated the importance of periodontal disease in the overall course of patients with leukemia suggests that such low-grade asymptomatic infections, while not life-threatening in the healthy patient, can become a major problem in patients who are myelosuppressed as a result of their disease or as a result of chemotherapy. Likewise, patients who have improperly fitting removable oral prostheses, who are constantly traumatizing their mucosa, are more likely to have mucosal breakdown during chemotherapy than other patients. There is no question that the level of oral care during treatment has a marked effect on the frequency and severity of oral complications of treatment. Patients in whom the level of gingival inflammation is minimized through scrupulous oral hygiene and those in whom debris is kept to a minimum have a reduced likelihood of developing either direct or indirect stomatotoxic effects of chemotherapy.

Therapy-related variables

Not all chemotherapeutic agents are equally stomatotoxic. Whereas drugs like methotrexate, Adriamycin, 5-fluorouracil, bleomycin, and cytosine arabinoside consistently cause stomatotoxicity, they do not all produce the same level of stomatotoxicity [1,6,13]. Other drugs may be rarely stomatotoxic. Generally, stomatotoxicity of the above agents is related to the total dose that the patient receives and the amount of time over which the patient receives the dose. In general, there is a direct relationship between dose and stomatotoxicity. However, if the total dose is given in increments rather than as a bolus, the toxic effects of the drugs may be minimized [14]. Concomitant therapy, such as radiation, occasionally has the effect of exaggerating chemotherapy-induced stomatotoxicity. This has been demonstrated in patients receiving both modalities of treatment for head and neck cancer; the frequency of mucositis is greater in patients receiving both chemotherapy and radiotherapy than in those receiving either modality of therapy alone [15].

Allogeneic bone-marrow transplantation is being used with increasing frequency in the treatment of the acute leukemias. This modality of therapy is discussed in detail in chapter 6. Approximately 1,600 marrow transplants are performed annually in about two dozen centers around the United States. Success has been achieved in patients with acute lymphocytic and acute nonlymphocytic leukemia and early studies suggest that patients with chronic myelogenous leukemia may be amenable to treatment. The rationale for this modality of therapy is to reconstitute the patient's hematopoietic system with normal, HLA-matched marrow following complete destruction of malignant cells. Approximately 40% of patients have appropriate donors. Destruction of the diseased myelogenous tissue is accomplished by a variety of chemotherapeutic agents and whole-body irradiation. Marrow transplants are most successfully obtained from an identical twin, although histocompatible family members are routinely used. Between the time the patient receives the graft and the time engraftment occurs, he/she is severely neutropenic and thrombocytopenic and is thus susceptible to infection and hemorrhage. Infections by bacteria, fungi, and viruses are a frequent and serious problem among patients receiving bone-marrow transplantation. A variety of techniques including protective environments, gastrointestinal sterilization, improved antibiotics, and granulocyte transfusions have been used with varying rates of success to reduce the frequency of early infections in these patients. Late infections, especially caused by viruses (herpes and cytomegaloviruses) remain a concern, although new antiviral agents may have significant antiherpes activity.

The oral cavity may be a significant factor in the success or failure of bone-marrow transplants in several ways. First, despite efforts to eliminate bacteria, numerous studies have documented the failure of antiinfective agents to sterilize the mouth [17]. The oral cavity thus harbors large numbers of bacteria, fungi, and viruses. Following loss of an intact epithelial barrier because of breakdown subsequent to chemotherapy, radiation, or preexisting oral disease, the affected tissue may become a significant portal of entry for these organisms. Second, thrombocytopenia coupled with breakdown of infected oral mucosa may result in significant hemorrhage in these patients. Finally, graft-versus-host reactions in which donor cells recognize and react against recipient tissue may produce acute and chronic changes in the mouth. The oral changes noted in acute graft-versus-host reactions are unresolved. However, more complete studies exist for chronic graft-versus-host reactions in which the sicca syndrome is a feature and has recently been attributed to destructive salivary gland ductal lesions [18]. Rampant caries similar to that noted in patients receiving radiotherapy may occur.

Premarrow transplant oral evaluation with elimination of all possible sources of infection is critical. Excellent oral hygiene, prophylactic antifungal and bacterial medication, and close follow-up are required to minimize oral morbidity associated with this procedure. Posttransplant care should include an aggressive anticaries protocol (chapter 7).

HISTOLOGIC CHANGES

In an effort to explain the clinical changes that occur in the mouth following chemotherapy, a number of histologic investigations have been performed. Animal studies, in which Shklar examined the mucosa of hamsters treated with methotrexate, demonstrated a high frequency of collagen degeneration [19]. In a study in humans treated with chemotherapy, Guggenheimer reported a high frequency of idiopathic atrophy in half of patients receiving treatment within three weeks of death [5]. Based on these observations, a mechanism for the development of direct stomatotoxicity was proposed in which reduced basal-cell mitosis produced decreased cell renewal and subsequent mucosal atrophy. The atrophic epithelium was then prone to secondary trauma, breakdown, and ulceration.

To further elucidate histologic mucosal changes associated with chemotherapy, Lockhart and Sonis examined 70 biopsy specimens taken from 20 cancer patients at autopsy [20]. Each patient had been recently treated with cancer chemotherapy which included at least one of the following: Adriamycin, cytoxin, and 5-fluorouracil. Patients with a variety of neoplasms were included in the study, although hematologic malignancies (leukemia and lymphoma) were the most common.

Epithelial hyperplasia and collagen degeneration were the most commonly observed changes and were noted in 75% of patients studied. Glandular degeneration, epithelial atrophy, and dysplasia were also frequent findings (figures 1–6 and 1–7). Histologic changes were most common in nonkeratinized mucosal surfaces. Changes tended to be either early, such as atrophy and dysplasia which occurred within two weeks of chemotherapy, or late, such as parakeratosis or glandular changes, which were not usually present until three weeks following treatment. It appeared that patients over age 50 had more atrophic changes than younger patients; this finding was consistent with earlier studies by Guggenheimer. Most histologic changes in mucosa occurred in patients who had chemotherapy within two weeks of death. This finding coincides with the turnover time of the oral mucosa (10 to 14 days) and suggests that beyond two weeks mucosal recovery may occur, as 40% of specimens examined at this time were normal.

Specimens were examined with respect to the patient's hematologic status. Specimens from patients with prolonged neutropenia had significantly more atrophic changes than specimens from nonneutropenic patients.

Degeneration of minor salivary glands was seen in half of all patients. Glandular changes, if they occurred to the same extent in the major salivary glands, may have contributed to the xerostomia seen frequently in patients receiving chemotherapy.

SUMMARY

The majority of oral complications of cancer chemotherapy occur as the direct effect of treatment on the oral mucosa or as a consequence of myelosuppression. Approximately 40% of patients who receive chemotherapy develop oral problems associated with each course of treatment. With the introduction of new drugs, higher dose schedules, and improved systemic management of myelosuppression, the scope of oral problems associated with chemotherapy is likely to increase. Both patient-related and therapy-related variables affect the frequency and severity of complications. These include patient age, type of malignancy, level of oral hygiene, dose, type and timing of treatment, and concommitant therapy. Early recognition and management of oral problems can significantly reduce their morbidity.

REFERENCES

1. Sonis ST, Sonis AL, Lieberman A: Oral complications in patients receiving treatment for malignancies other than of the head and neck. J Am Dent Assoc 97:468–472, 1978.
2. Sonis AT, Sonis ST: Oral complications of cancer chemotherapy in pediatric patients. J Pedodontics 3:122–128, 1979.
3. Dreizen S, Bodey GP, Brown LR: Opportunistic gram-negative bacillary infections in leukemia. Oral manifestations during myelosuppression. Postgrad Med 55:133–139, 1974.
4. The EORTC International Antimicrobial Therapy Project Group: Three antibiotic regimens in the treatment of infection in febrile granulocytopenic patients with cancer. J Infect Dis 137:14–29, 1978.
5. Guggenheimer J, Verbin RS, Appel BN, Schmitz J: Clinicopathologic effects of cancer chemotherapeutic agents on human buccal mucosa. Oral Surg 44:58–63, 1977.
6. Lockhart PB, Sonis ST: Relationship of oral complications to peripheral blood leukocyte and platelet counts in patients receiving cancer chemotherapy. Oral Surg 48:21–28, 1979.
7. Bodey GP: Oral manifestations of the myeloproliferative diseases. Postgrad Med 49:115–121, 1971.
8. Lynch MA, Ship II: Initial oral manifestations of leukemia. J Am Dent Assoc 75:932–940, 1967.
9. Stafford RF, Lockhart PB, Sonis AL, Sonis ST: Hematologic parameters as predictors of oral involvement in the presentation of acute leukemia. J Oral Med 37:38–41, 1982.

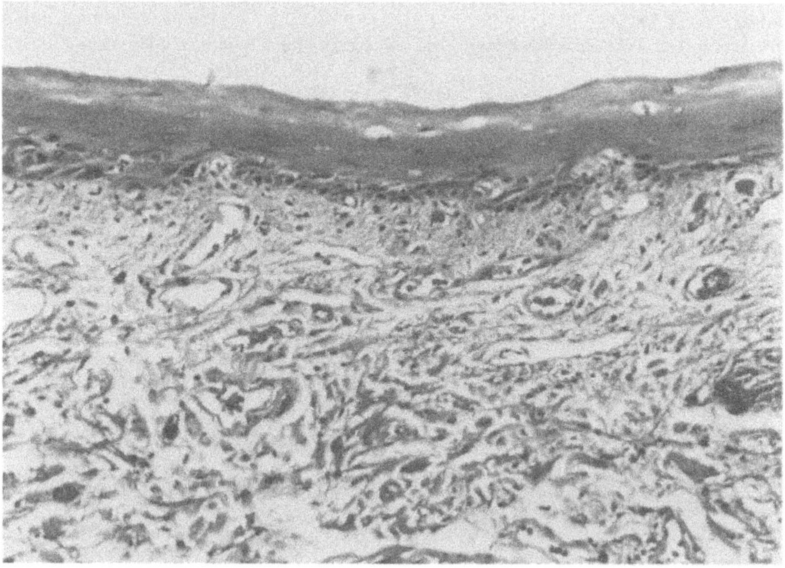

Figure 1–6. Histologic section from the labial mucosa of a 68-year-old male who received chemotherapy 12 days prior to death. Note epithelial thinning and atrophy and marked collagen degeneration (H + E × 300). (Lockhart and Sonis, J Dermatol Surg Oncol 7:1021, 1981.)

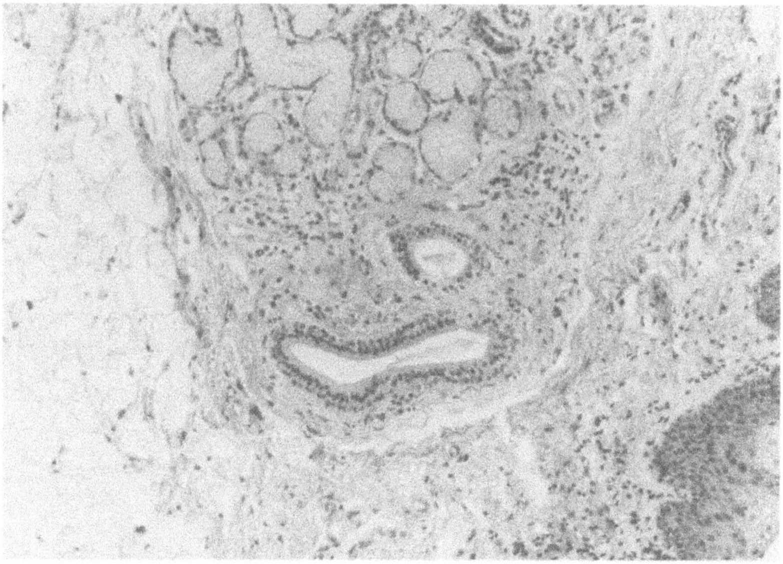

Figure 1–7. Histologic section from the tongue of a patient with lymphoma. Note glandular changes and evidence of epithelial atrophy (H + E × 300).

10. Sonis AL, Sonis ST: Gingival crevice lymphoblasts in children with acute lymphoblastic leukemia. J Periodontol 52:276–279, 1981.
11. Barakat NJ, Toto PD, Choukas NC: Aging and cell renewal of oral epithelium. J Periodontol, 40:599–602, 1969.
12. Overholser D, Peterson D, Williams L, Schimpff S: Periodontal infection in patients with acute nonlymphocytic leukemia: Prevalence of acute exacerbation. Arch Intern Med 142:551–554, 1982.
13. Dreizen S, Bodey GP, Rodriguez V: Oral complications of cancer chemotherapy. Postgrad Med 58:95–82, 1975.
14. Volger W, Huguley C, and Kerr W: Toxicity and antitumor effect of divided doses of methotrexate. Arch Intern Med. 115:285–293, 1965.
15. Archibald D: Personal Communication.
16. Thomas ED, et al.: Bone marrow transplantation. N Engl J Med 292:895–902, 1975.
17. Brown LR, Dreizen S, Bodey GP: Effect of immunosuppression on the human oral flora. In *Comparative Immunology of the Oral Cavity,* Mergenhagen, SE Scherp HW (eds), DHEW Publication (NIH) 73–438, 1973, pp. 204–220.
18. Sale GE, Shulman HM, Schubert MM, Sullivan KM, Kopecky KJ, Hackman RC, Morton TH, Szorb R, Thomas ED: Oral and ophthalmic pathology of graft versus host disease in man: predictive value of the lip biopsy. Hum Pathol 12:1022–1030, 1981.
19. Shklar G: The effect of 4-amino-N^{10}-methyl-pterogl-glutamine acid on oral mucosa of experimental animals. J Oral Ther Pharmacol 4:374–377, 1968.
20. Lockhart PB, Sonis ST: Alterations in the oral mucosa caused by chemotherapeutic agents. J Dermatol Surg Oncol 7:1019–1025, 1981.

2. PHARMACOLOGY OF CHEMOTHERAPEUTIC AGENTS

NICHOLAS R. BACHUR, M.D., Ph.D.

INTRODUCTION

During the recorded history of mankind, we have continually sought cures to our ills. This quest has included search for a magic bullet, a substance or chemical that will relieve us of our cancers. The first sustained efforts in the discovery of anticancer drugs began just 40 years ago, with the clinical trials of nitrogen mustards and alkylating agents [1,2]. This coincided with the entrance of the biological sciences into a Golden Era, a time when fundamental life processes were being explained and understood in chemical and physical terms. With the elucidation of cellular metabolic pathways and metabolites came the design and development of antimetabolites such as the antifolates [3]. Other classes of chemotherapeutic agents evolved until the rate of development doubled in the early 1960s. This doubling of anticancer-drug discoveries was the result of increased governmental funding for research, the increased search for substances with anticancer activity, and the development of new methods for drug screening such as new transplantable animal tumors to screen for active drugs [4].

This history of the chemotherapeutic management of cancer has not been studded with successes that have marked the development and use of immunological and antibacterial agents against microbial infections. With infectious illnesses, treatment is aimed at a foreign invader—a microbe that has a different identity from the host and is vulnerable due to this difference. Antimicrobial drugs can be designed to interfere with microbial metabolic pathways and cellular functions that do not exist or are relatively unimportant in mammalian cells. The antimicrobial drug therefore has a high degree of selectivity since the microbes are highly vulnerable to the drug but the host cells are not.

D.E. Peterson and S.T. Sonis (eds.), ORAL COMPLICATIONS OF CANCER CHEMOTHERAPY, 13-22.

Designing a drug to kill or selectively inhibit the cancer cell is a very different task. The cancer cell is self. It is a descendant of normal host cells and is nearly identical to those cells. Little opportunity is available for a drug to act selectively on a cancer cell in the animal. Nevertheless, there is a selectivity; otherwise, no drugs would be successful. The fact that anticancer drugs can selectively kill cancer cells in an animal or a human indicates that cancer cells are more sensitive to drug action than are normal cells of the host.

Much of the selectivity of cell kill by drugs relates to the cellular DNA target since most anticancer drugs kill cells by directly affecting the cellular DNA itself or the molecular events leading to DNA synthesis and replication. Therefore, cells undergoing growth and division are more sensitive to these drugs than cells that are in resting phase. Since cancer cells and normal cells divide at similar rates, individual cell division is not a factor in the selectivity of drugs for the malignant cells. When taken as an entire population of cells, however, tumor tissue has a larger growth fraction than normal tissue. That is, the percentage of cells undergoing cellular growth and division in tumor tissue is larger than the percentage in normal tissue. This disparity in growth fractions presents the opportunity for selectivity of drug action since a larger percentage of tumor cells will be at risk to drug action than normal cells at any one time.

As a result of quantitative studies with mouse tumors, scientists have shown that various drugs or anticancer agents affect tumor and normal cells in different ways [5]. There is a selectivity of action against dividing cells by some agents (cell-cycle specific) whereas other drugs kill both dividing cells and nondividing cells (cell-cycle nonspecific). Drugs and agents have therefore been assigned a classification for their selectivities of action (table 2–1). Agents in class I (e.g., radiation, alkylating agents) show no differential selectivity and kill cells in all phases of their replication cycle. Agents in class II (e.g., vinblastine, amethopterin) show a 500-fold selectivity for murine lymphoma and kill cells in one segment of the cell's replication cycle. Class III agents (e.g., actinomycin D, cyclophosphamide) have a 10,000-fold selectivity against murine lymphoma cells and appear to kill cells in all phases of cellular replication.

In human malignancies, the selectivity of anticancer agents against a tumor may be quite small. However, by careful planning of treatment regimens, the correct combination of surgery, radiotherapy, and chemotherapy, and the correct selection of drug combinations, small selectivities can be amplified to yield a successful therapeutic result.

CLASSES OF DRUGS

The anticancer drugs are divided into classes based on their source or mode of drug action. The major classes are alkylating agents, antimetabolites, natural products, hormones, and miscellaneous substances (table 2–2).

Alkylating agents are very reactive substances that form chemical bonds with target molecules in the cell [6]. These important target molecules are DNA, RNA, and protein. By forming chemical bonds with nucleophilic groups of the target molecules, alkylating drugs react with and modify the internal cellular components to such a degree that the cell is either killed or prevented from replicating. Double-armed alkylating agents may cross-link between DNA strands and nucleophilic groups of other macromolecules. Although

Table 2–1. Classification of chemotherapeutic agents by the dose-survival curves obtained for colony-forming cells exposed to the agents for 24 hours in vivo

Class of Agent	Agents Assigned	Survival Curves Obtained	Suggested Action at the Cellular Level
I	γ Radiation Nitrogen mustard	Exponential, with similar sensitivity for normal hematopoietic and lymphoma colony-forming cells	Agents kill cells in all portions of the generation cycle. Sensitivity not a marked function of proliferative state of the cells
II	H^3-thymidine Vinblastine Amethopterin Azaserine	Decrease to a constant saturation value at high doses. Lymphoma colony-forming cells are much less sensitive than normal hematopoietic colony-forming cells	Agents kill cells in only one portion of the generation cycle. Cells not entering this portion during the period of exposure survive
III	5-Fluorouracil Actinomycin D Cyclophosphamide	Exponential, with sensitivity of lymphoma colony-forming cells much greater than normal hematopoietic colony-forming cells. No saturation at the doses employed	Agents kill cells in all or most portions of the generation cycle. Sensitivity of cell population depends strongly on the fraction in the proliferative state
Unassigned	6-Mercaptopurine Hydrocortisone	May be II or III Little effect on survival of either normal or lymphoma colony-forming cells	

Source: Bruce WR, Meeker BE, Valeriote FA: Comparison of the sensitivity of normal hematopoietic and transplanted lymphoma colony-forming cells to chemotherapeutic agents administered *in vivo*. J Natl Cancer Inst 37:233–245, 1966.

other cellular molecules may also serve as the target site for chemical reaction by alkylating agents, the replicative activity of DNA in both RNA and DNA synthesis appears to be the most sensitive reactive site for alkylating activity. Most alkylating drugs can react immediately upon administration to the patient; however, some commonly used drugs such as cyclophosphamide are specifically designed to require metabolic activation by the patient's liver enzymes before they become active as antitumor agents [7]. Subclassifications of alkylating drugs include: (1) nitrogen mustards; (2) nitrosoureas; (3) ethylenimines; (4) triazines; and (5) alkyl sulfonates.

Antimetabolites were among the earliest of antitumor agents discovered and are in extensive clinical use today. These drugs are structurally similar to natural metabolic intermediates of cellular macromolecules; by substituting for the natural metabolite, normal metabolism is therefore blocked. These drugs are especially effective against cells that are undergoing rapid metabolism or cell division. Antimetabolites consist primarily of analogs of: (1) folic acid; (2) purine; and (3) pyrimidine.

Methotrexate is the most well known and most frequently used folic acid analog; this drug acts by inhibiting the enzyme dihydrofolate reductase, thereby interfering with one-carbon-transfer reactions. Since one-carbon-transfer reactions are important processes

Table 2–2. Anticancer drugs

Alkylating agents
Nitrogen mustards
Nitrosoureas
Ethylenimines
Triazines
Alkyl sulfonates
Antimetabolites
Folic acid analogs
Purine analogs
Pyrimidine analogs
Natural products
Antibiotics
Actinomycins
Anthracyclines
Bleomycins
Mitomycins
Mithramycins
Vinca alkaloids
Enzymes-asparaginase
Hormones
Miscellaneous
Hydroxyurea
Procarbazine
Cis-platinum
Mitotane
Radioactive isotopes

in the cellular synthesis of nucleic acids, folic acid analogs interfere with the building of nucleic acids and ultimately the synthesis of DNA, RNA, and protein [8].

Both purines and pyrimidines are nucleic acid building blocks for the macromolecular DNA and RNA. Therefore, if antimetabolites are designed as imitation pyrimidines or purines, they can interfere with the biosynthesis and functioning of DNA and RNA. Purine analogs (e.g., 6-mercaptopurine or thioguanine) and pyrimidine analogs (e.g. 5-fluorouracil and cytosine arabinoside) function in this fashion [9,10].

In the search for anticancer drugs, a large number of naturally occurring products from tree, plant, fungal, mold, microbial, and tissue extracts have been screened against transferable mouse tumors. From these natural substances have come some of the most effective anticancer drugs: (1) very potent antibiotics; (2) the vinca alkaloids; and (3) the enzyme asparaginase.

The antibiotic subgroup of microbial products includes: (1) actinomycins (actinomycin D); (2) anthracyclines (doxorubicin, daunorubicin); (3) bleomycin; (4) mitomycin C; and (5) mithramycin. These antibiotics have widely varied chemical structures and characteristics; however, they all act by binding to cellular DNA and interfering with the biochemical processing, replication, and transcription of the DNA. Nevertheless, the intracellular actions of these antibiotics are quite complex and go beyond simple binding to DNA. Each antibiotic type has specific binding characteristics for DNA; some antibiotics require cellular enzymes for activation and others bind to metal ions as part of their interactions with DNA.

While their effects on cellular processes vary, evidence is accumulating that many antibiotics are involved in cellular electron transport whereby free radicals are formed, contributing to their cytotoxic action [11–14].

The vinca alkaloids vinblastine and vincristine are natural products from periwinkle plants. These complex structures inhibit cellular mitosis by binding to critical microtubular protein structures and disrupting the mitotic spindle apparatus. Also among the natural products is the enzyme L-asparaginase, which has been used to produce selective starvation of malignant cells by limiting the availability of the essential amino acid asparagine to malignant cells.

Hormones, although primarily natural products, are considered separately because of their unique action. They retain important positions as therapeutic drugs for several types of malignancies. The adrenocorticosteroid prednisone is used in the therapy of acute and chronic lymphocytic leukemias, lymphomas, and breast tumors. The mechanism of action is unknown. In the sex-linked cancers of the prostate, breast, endometrium, and so on, progestins, estrogens, and androgens can be effective for inhibiting tumor growth, but they are not curative.

The miscellaneous group of anticancer agents encompasses a wide spectrum of agents. Examples are hydroxyurea, procarbazine, cisplatin, mitotane, radioactive isotopes such as phosphorus^{32}, gold^{138}, and iodine^{131}, and others. Although the miscellaneous group does not fit a specific mode of action, members of this group are very useful clinically against specific tumor types. For example, hydroxyurea is useful in chronic granulocytic leukemia, and cisplatin has shown activity against testicular tumors. Also, a class of agents called radiosensitizing agents, which act to increase cellular sensitivity to ionizing radiation, has been recently undergoing clinical trial. Finally, additional research is being continually conducted to make anticancer agents more selective by linking the drug to a carrier molecule. The carrier molecule is designed or selected because it has a higher affinity for the cancer cell than for normal cells.

UTILIZATION OF CHEMOTHERAPEUTIC AGENTS

Clinical trials are used to analyze effectiveness and toxicity in humans. After the phase I or dosage determination and preliminary human toxicity trials of a new experimental drug, the drug is tested in varying regimens against different types of cancers in humans. From these phase II and phase III clinical trials, recommended dosage regimens and therapeutic guidelines are developed in which drug activities against cancers are described. Ultimately, the selection of therapy for any patient is determined by several factors, including tumor type, tumor burden, cell-cycle considerations, health, age, and performance status of the patient, as well as his/her immunocompetence.

To utilize chemotherapy adequately, an understanding of cell-growth kinetics and cell biology is essential. Cells progress through stages of development while they are synthesizing, growing, and dividing. However, most cells in the body are fully developed and differentiated and are no longer cycling and replicating. A portion of normal cells in tissues undergoing cellular turnover are in the process of controlled growth and division (e.g., skin, bone marrow, gastrointestinal tract, and so on). In contrast, tumor cells continue to grow and divide beyond the normal control of the host. The stages of cell growth and division

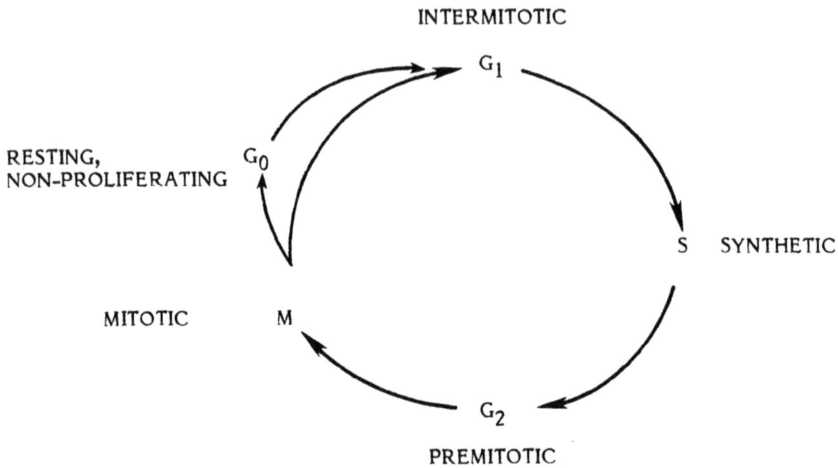

Figure 2–1. A cell in the G_0 phase can progress through the cell-proliferation cycle by entering the G_1 phase. Once proliferation begins, the process is irreversible until the developing cell proceeds through M (mitosis) and two cells emerge. These may then move into G_0 or proceed into G_1 for continued proliferation.

are called the cell cycle (figure 2–1). Cells begin the cell cycle in the intermitotic phase, or G_1. Elements necessary for cell growth and division are produced in the synthetic or S phase. During this phase DNA, RNA, and major protein synthesis occurs. At the cessation of S phase, the premitotic or G_2 phase occurs, followed by M phase or mitosis. Cells that are not in the replicating cycle move into the G_0 or nonproliferating phase, from which they may return to the active proliferating phase. Since the S phase is the period when the cell carries out intensive metabolic and synthetic activities, it is the phase when the cell may be most sensitive to agents that interfere with DNA, RNA, and protein synthesis.

With the current selection of agents, the physician can plan chemotherapy to eradicate the maximal number of cancer cells. As noted previously, drugs may act at different points and by different mechanisms in the cell cycle and can be selected partly on this basis. In rapidly growing tumors where the cellular doubling time is short, the cells move through the cell cycle more frequently and may be more susceptible to well-timed chemotherapy. For example, rapidly growing tumors such as lymphomas, choriocarcinoma, and some types of leukemia show increased susceptibility to chemotherapy, whereas tumors with long doubling time may be treated more effectively by irradiation or surgery followed by chemotherapy (table 2–3).

Dosage scheduling of the drugs is important to formulate the most efficient means of killing the cancer cells by chemotherapy. Using leukemic mouse models, it has been shown that timing of administration of anticancer drugs is critical to killing adequate numbers of the dividing tumor cells [15]. Cell kill occurs on a fixed percentile basis (first order), so the spacing of administration of the drug, as well as the amount of drug given to the maximum tolerated dose where toxicity is limiting, is very important. For example, a drug may kill 99.9% of malignant cells, but if the tumor cells number 10^{10} (approximately 10

Table 2–3. Kinetic parameters of some human tumors

Type	Doubling Time (days)	Labeling Index (%)	Growth Fraction (%)	Cell Loss (%)	Daily Turnover Rate (%)
Embryonal tumors	27 (76)	30 (30)	90	93	49
Lymphomas	29 (41)	29 (15)	90	93	47
Sarcomas	41 (87)	4 (32)	11	68	5.5
Squamous carcinomas	58 (51)	8 (68)	25	89	10
Adenocarcinomas	83 (134)	2 (121)	6	71	2

Source: Tubiana M, Malaise EP: Growth rate and cell kinetics in human tumours: some pragmatic and therapeutic implications. In *Scientific Foundations of Oncology,* Symington T, Carter RL (eds), Chicago, Year Book Publishers, 1976, pp. 126–136.
(As adapted by Hellman S, DeVita VT. Principles of cancer biology: kinetics of cellular proliferation. In *Cancer—Principles and Practice of Oncology,* DeVita VT, Hellman S, Rosenberg SA (eds), Philadelphia, JB Lippincott Co, 1982, p 77.)

gm tumor), 10^7 (10 mg tumor) cells survive a single treatment. Theoretically, a well-timed repetitive treatment schedule can further deplete the remaining cells in 99.9% kill cycles until the last remaining tumor cell is eliminated (figure 2–2).

Research into the behavior and biology of malignant cells has established principles in the understanding of tumor cell growth, mutation rate, and population kinetics. There is a definite inverse relationship between the tumor cell burden or the size of the tumor at the start of treatment and the survival of the animal or patient. Thus the chemotherapy-induced cell kill is enhanced if the size of the tumor is smaller when chemotherapy is started. For this reason, the debulking of tumors by surgery or radiation therapy is useful. Also, smaller tumors have a higher growth fraction than large tumors. As a result, a larger percentage of their cells are replicating and are susceptible to chemotherapeutic agents. As the tumor size increases the growth slows and the cells are less likely to be in the susceptible cell cycle phase. Resting cells are resistant to most agents.

Since tumor cells are nearly identical to normal cells, anticancer drugs will express activity (i.e., toxicity) against normal tissues as well as tumor tissues. Those normal tissues that are most susceptible and sensitive are those undergoing proliferation, such as the bone marrow, the gastrointestinal tract (including the oral mucosa), the hair follicles, gonads, and tissues that are undergoing repair (wound healing). Other organs that may also be affected by the chemotherapeutic agents for other reasons include liver, central nervous system, heart, lung, kidney and skin.

With bone-marrow suppression, the production of blood cells decreases, leading to leukopenia, anemia, and thrombocytopenia. Myelosuppressed patients are often extremely susceptible to infection since they have decreased functional leukocytes and immunoglobulin production is impaired because of suppressed lymphocytes. Since platelet formation is inhibited, bleeding and hemorrhage becomes a major problem. Bone-marrow toxicity is generally the most important dose-limiting factor. Since the human bone marrow can recover from the toxic effects of chemotherapy in about three weeks, treatment scheduling of chemotherapy is based on 21-day intervals to allow the bone marrow to recover.

Other organs may also be profoundly affected. The gastrointestinal tract may develop oral ulceration, intestinal ulceration, and infection, with associated pain and diarrhea. Hair growth may be suppressed and alopecia may result. Gonadal function may be inhibited, resulting in menstrual irregularities, amenorrhea, and infertility. Altered tissue repair,

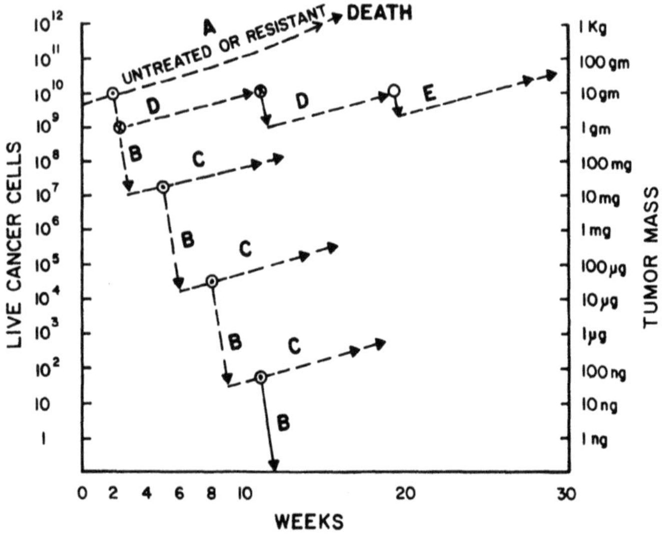

Figure 2–2. Representation of tumor growth and tumor response to chemotherapy.

A. Growth of untreated or drug-resistant tumor leading to death of host
B. Treatment cycles yielding 99.9% cell kill
C. Regrowth of tumor after 99.9% cell kill
D. Regrowth of tumor after 90% cell kill
E. Regrowth of tumor after 80% cell kill showing resistance developing

Source: Skipper HE, Schabel FM, Wilcox WS: Experimental evaluation of potential anticancer agents. XIII. On the criteria and kinetics associated with "curability" of experimental leukemia. Cancer Chemo Rep 35(1): 1–111, 1964.

including healing of surgical wounds, may result. Rapid destruction of the tumor mass itself may yield by-products that are toxic to the patient.

In planning a patient's chemotherapy, the physician must determine that adequate elimination of drugs from the patient will occur; otherwise, excessive toxicity may develop. For drugs in which hepatobiliary excretion is important, liver function and biliary flow must be adequate. Similarly, for drugs excreted in urine, kidney function must be normal. Retention of the drug or active metabolites may result in higher levels of the drug than is desired. In the case that impaired excretion is present, appropriately lowered dosage of the drug may be administered.

Adequate drug therapy must be given a patient to ensure optimum tumor-cell kill on the first therapeutic attempt. Through animal studies, the dosage and tissue or plasma concentrations of drug necessary to kill susceptible tumor cells have often been established. Therefore the dosage of a drug to a patient is determined by the CXT (drug concentration times exposure time) that is necessary to obtain a tumor toxic plasma drug concentration. The individual dosage of drug and the frequency of its administration will be determined by the tumor type as well as the patient's diagnosis and overall status. Despite the toxicity resultant from chemotherapy, therapy will not be effective unless virtually all tumor cells are eliminated. By using less than tumor cytotoxic drug dosage, the chance of developing drug resistance in the tumor is increased. Only drugs that are effective against the tumor being treated must be used since ineffective drugs only yield toxicity in the patient.

By combining drugs in the treatment regimen, malignant cells can be attacked by agents with different mechanisms of action [16]. This can produce a higher cell kill and also allow fewer resistant cells to develop. In the design of combination chemotherapy, the following principals are used:

1. Only drugs active against the specific malignancy in question are used.
2. Drugs with different mechanisms of action are combined to effect higher kill rate.
3. Drugs with minimally overlapping toxicities are selected to reduce the toxicity to the patient.
4. Drugs are used at their optimal dosage and scheduling.
5. Repeated drug administration is done as frequently as possible to the limit of toxicity.

Important advances that have occurred in the cancer treatment by chemotherapy have been: (1) the use of intermittent high-dose chemotherapy to allow the patient's bone marrow to recover between drug courses; (2) the use of rescue therapy (e.g., antidotal methotrexate therapy) for the protection of normal cells; (3) the use of combination chemotherapy to yield greater killing of the cancer cells and less toxicity to the patient; and (4) the use of drugs as adjuvants to surgery, radiation therapy, or both to eliminate micrometastatic cancer that is not clinically evident when the primary tumor is treated.

Notable chemotherapeutic successes include Burkett's lymphoma, choriocarcinoma, acute lymphocytic leukemia of childhood, Hodgkin's disease, lymphosarcoma, embryonal testicular carcinoma, Wilms' tumor, rhabdomyosarcoma, and retinoblastoma. Progress continues to be made in the therapy of small-cell cancer of the lung and breast cancer. However, significant effectiveness of chemotherapy is lacking for many malignancies. With the continued development of more effective and less toxic drugs as well as a better understanding of the biological basis of malignancy, scientists will combine these practical and basic research approaches for curative anticancer therapy.

SUMMARY

Chemotherapy is widely used in the treatment of many types of cancer. However, considerable side effects often result due to the relative nonspecificity of the drugs. Positive clinical results can often be achieved by using carefully selected combinations of drugs or by using chemotherapy in conjunction with other modes of therapy.

REFERENCES

1. Adair FE, Bagg HJ: Experimental and clinical studies on the treatment of cancer by dichlorethylsulphide (mustard gas). Ann Surg 93:190–199, 1931.
2. Gilman A, Philips FS: The biological actions and therapeutic applications of the B-chloroethyl amines and sulfides. Science 103 (2675): 409–415, 1946.
3. Farber S, Diamond LK, Mercer RD, Sylvester RF, Wolff JA: Temporary remissions in acute leukemia in children produced by folic acid antagonist, 4-aminopteroyl-glutamic acid (aminopterin). N Engl J Med 238 (23): 787–793, 1948.

4. Frei E: Combination cancer therapy: presidential address. Cancer Res 32(12): 2593–2607, 1972.
5. Bruce WR, Meeker BE, Valeriote FA: Comparison of the sensitivity of normal hematopoietic and transplanted lymphoma colony-forming cells to chemotherapeutic agents administered *in vivo*. J Natl Cancer Inst 37(2): 233–245, 1966.
6. Price CC: Chemistry of alkylation. In *Antineoplastic and immunosuppressive agents, part II,* Sartorelli AC, Johns DG (eds), Berlin, Springer-Verlag, 1975, pp 1–5.
7. Foley GE, Friedman OM, Drolet BP: Studies on the mechanism of action of Cytoxan—evidence of activation *in vivo* and *in vitro*. Cancer Res 21(1): 57–70, 1961.
8. Bertino JR: Folate antagonists as chemotherapeutic agents. Ann NY Acad Sci 186:5–6, 1971.
9. Burchenal JH, Ellison RR: Symposium on the experimental pharmacology and clinical use of antimetabolites Part IX. The pyrimidine and purine antagonists. Clin Pharmacol Ther 2(4): 523–541, 1961.
10. Heidelberger C: Fluorinated pyrimidines. Prog Nucleic Acid Res Mol Biol 4:1–50, 1965.
11. DeMarco A, Arcamone F, Zunimo FG: Biological activity and mechanism of action. In: *Antibiotics III. Mechanism of action of antimicrobial and antitumor agents,* Corcoran JW, Hahn FE (eds), Berlin, Springer-Verlag, 1975, pp 101–128.
12. Kersten H: Mechanism of action of mitomycins. In *Antineoplastic and immunosuppressed agents Part II,* Sartorelli AC, Johns DG (eds), Berlin, Springer-Verlag, 1975, pp 47–64.
13. Blum RH, Carter SK, Agre K: A clinical review of Bleomycin—a new antineoplastic agent. Cancer 31 (4): 903–914, 1973.
14. Bachur NR, Gordon SL, Gee MV: A general mechanism for microsomal activation of quinone anticancer agents to free radicals. Cancer Res 38 (6):1745–1750, 1978.
15. Skipper HE, Schabel FM, Wilcox WS: Experimental evaluation of potential anticancer agents. XIII. On the criteria and kinetics associated with "curability" of experimental leukemia. Cancer Chemo Rep 35(1): 1–111, 1964.
16. DeVita VT, Young RC, Canellos GP: Combination versus single agent chemotherapy: a review of the basis for selection of drug treatment of cancer. Cancer 35 (1):98–110, 1975.

3. PRINCIPLES OF INFECTION MANAGEMENT AND PREVENTION

JOSEPH AISNER, M.D.
STEPHEN C. SCHIMPFF, M.D.

INTRODUCTION

Infection among patients with cancer, particularly those receiving myelosuppressive or immunosuppressive treatment, has become an area of concern for all members of the health care delivery system involved in the care of these patients. In recent years there has evolved a body of knowledge relevant to the treatment and prevention of infectious complications that has given many cancer patients the opportunity to benefit from more aggressive chemotherapy, surgery, radiation therapy, or combined modality treatments [1]. Concomitant progress has also been made in other aspects of supportive care such as cell component therapy which has contributed to the improvement in the useful lives of many cancer patients [2]. Despite these many gains in supportive care, infection remains the leading cause of morbidity and mortality [1]. This severe morbidity and high mortality caused by opportunistic pathogens requires a basic understanding of the epidemiology of these infections as well as a systematic approach to diagnosis and treatment. In addition, there is a constant evolution in the type and site of infection involved so that all members of the health care delivery team must be cognizant of these factors to bring maximal knowledge into the management of infections in the cancer patient [3]. The purpose of this chapter is to review the approach to infection in these patients that is, the compromised host, and enable members of the health profession team to recognize and deal with the predisposing factors, gain familiarity with sites of infections, and develop a rational systematic approach to the diagnosis, treatment, and prevention of such infections.

D.E. Peterson and S.T. Sonis (eds.), ORAL COMPLICATIONS OF CANCER CHEMOTHERAPY, 23-40.

FACTORS LEADING TO INFECTION

The types of infections and the sites at which they occur may vary widely in accordance with the predisposing factors present. Virtually by definition, the patient with cancer undergoing myelosuppressive or immunosuppressive treatment is a compromised host by nature of the underlying disease, the treatment, or both [4]. Thus the patient with a marrow failure state such as acute leukemia may have one set of infectious complications [4,5], the patient with lymphoma receiving irradiation or chemotherapy or both may have a different set of infectious complications [4], whereas patients undergoing various organ transplantation may have yet different types of infection [6,7]. Among the most important predisposing conditions are the status of marrow function, the immunologic status, obstructive phenomena, and various iatrogenic procedures (table 3–1).

Granulocytopenia, whether due to underlying disease or treatment or both, is a major predisposing factor to both bacterial and fungal infections. The association of the degree of granulocytopenia and the incidence of infection was first defined by Bodey and associates in patients with acute leukemia [8]. This study showed that as the absolute granulocyte count dropped below 1,000/μl, the incidence and severity of infection rose. Further studies have clearly demonstrated that the incidence of severe infection and bacteremia rises markedly as the absolute granulocyte count falls below 100/μl with a dramatic increase in the incidence of infection per time at risk (figure 3–1) below this level [9]. This association is important because the intensity of treatments for many solid tumors regularly produces significant neutropenia. In addition, certain diseases such as acute leukemia, aplastic anemia, and certain organ transplantations have essential failure of the marrow to produce myeloid cells because of disease or treatment or both. In these cases the duration of severe neutropenia may last three or more weeks. Generally, patients with many lymphomas and most solid tumors have shorter periods of neutropenia because the therapy is designed and modified to produce a mild transient nadir of the leukocyte count. Recently, however, more aggressive therapy has been advanced for many tumors and the duration of neutro-

Table 3–1. Factors that predispose to the development of infection in the cancer patient

Underlying disease
Marrow failure states
Disease
Treatment
Immunologic deficiences
Disease
Treatment
Granulocytopenia
Immune deficiences
Cellular
Humoral
Obstruction
Damage to mucosal and integumental barriers
Iatrogenic procedures
Acquisition of new organisms

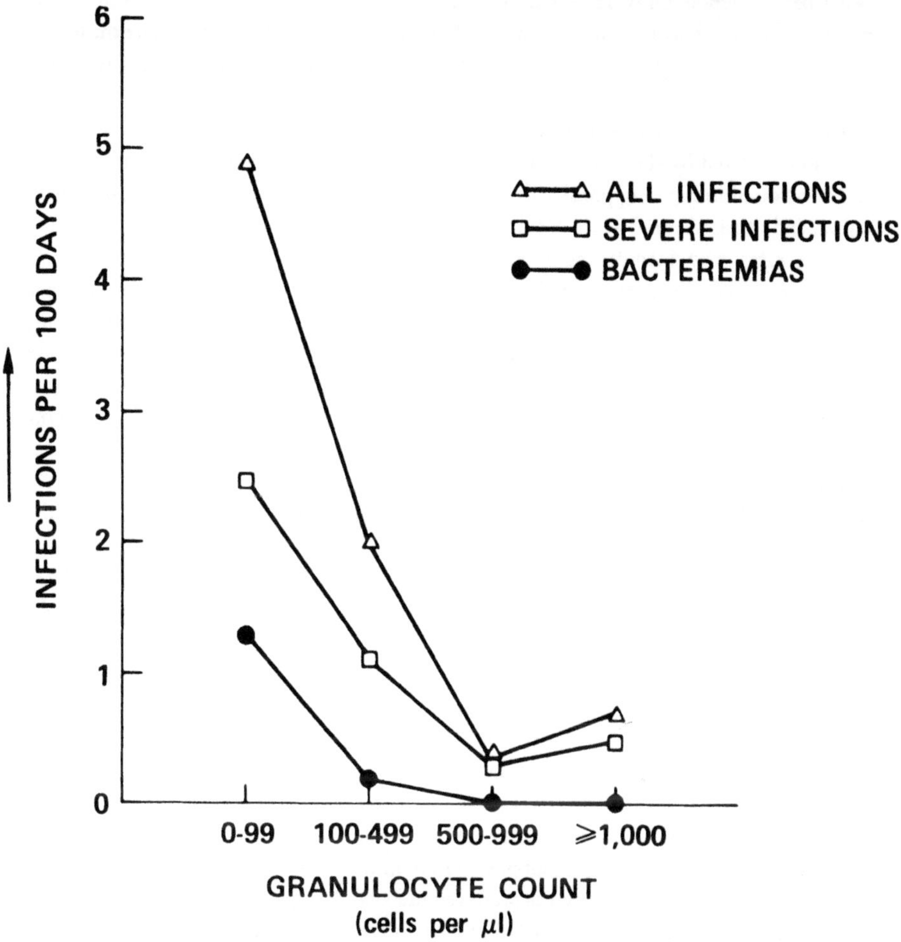

Figure 3–1. Graphic relationship between absolute granulocyte count and incidence of infection per 100 days of risk. The incidence of infection increases with the reduction in absolute granulocyte count. Most important increase in severe infections and bacteremias occur when absolute granulocyte falls below 500/μ 1. Data based on 64 newly diagnosed patients with acute nonlymphocytic leukemia given intensive combination chemotherapy at the University of Maryland Cancer Center (formerly BCRC) between 1974–1977. Source: Reproduced from Schimpff SC, Infection in the immunocompromised host. Mandell, Douglass, Bennett (eds), *Principles and Practice of Infectious Diseases,* with permission of John Wiley and Sons.

penia has correspondingly increased. Thus the model for the treatment of neutropenia-related infections remains acute leukemia and similar marrow failure states where the lessons and technology have produced potential applications to other cancer treatment situations [10].

Patients with immune deficiencies usually have specific bacterial, fungal, and viral infections dictated by the cell-mediated or humoral deficits and dependent upon intensity and duration of immunosuppressive therapy, thymic dysplasia, Hodgkin's disease, transplantation, and other treatments, are examples of cell-mediated immune deficiencies. Infections in these cases may include those caused by *Listeria monocytogenes, Toxoplasma gondii, Cryptococcus neoformans,* or the varicella zoster virus [11]. Patients with humoral immune defects such as multiple myeloma, chronic lymphocytic leukemia, or functional asplenia tend to have infections for which antibody appears to be the major source of infection prevention. Infections in such circumstances are frequently caused by encapsulated organisms that evoke humoral antibody, such as *Streptococcus pneumoniae* and *Hemophilus influenzae* [11,12]. In both circumstances the immune system may be disturbed while the inflammatory response is intact. However, it is also possible that disease, therapy, or both have produced both myeloid and immune suppression; in these circumstances, the host has the added risk associated with granulocytopenia.

Obstructive phenomena can predispose to infection in virtually any setting and are particularly common in tumors that occlude natural passages. Examples include postobstructive urinary tract infection or ascending cholangitis due to biliary obstruction. A complex problem arises when obstructive phenomena complicate other predisposing factors such as granulocytopenia or immune deficiencies, in light of the increased susceptibility to a wide variety of organisms as well as the problems associated with the need for invasive procedures required to relieve the obstruction.

Chemotherapy, radiation therapy, or both can produce damage to the mucosa and skin which are natural barriers protecting the body from microbial invasion. Thus the settings of immunosuppression and myelosuppression are greatly enhanced as factors predisposing to infection when cancer therapy has produced mucosal damage of the mouth, esophagous, or other areas of the alimentary canal. Similarly, breaks of the integument such as trauma, surgery, or other invasive procedures allow migration of organisms across these natural body barriers.

This underscores the large number of potentially predisposing iatrogenically induced infections due to medical and surgical procedures. For example, insertions of indwelling intravenous or urinary catheters can increase the occurrence of nosocomial infections. The introduction of endoscopes [13,14] or the manipulation of body surfaces such as scaling the teeth or irrigating the gums [15] can result in transient bacteremia in normal individuals and can cause iatrogenic infection in the setting of other predisposing factors.

Finally, another important area in the predisposition of infection relates to the acquisition and colonization of various body areas such as mouth, skin, urinary and gastrointestinal tracts with refractory or antibiotic resistant organisms, particularly those acquired within the hospital. Many studies have clearly demonstrated that patients become infected with the organisms that they harbor or acquire [10,12]; thus the acquisition of a resistant organism or a secondary organism (even of low virulence) in the compromised host can lead to significant infection [16]. This forms an important rationale for infection-prevention methods practiced by all health providers.

Despite the diversity of the predisposing factors to infection in the cancer patient, generally those specific factors pertinent to any given patient are few and easily summarized by a review of the patient's status with regard to granulocytopenia, immune function, obstructive phenomena, damage to natural barriers, iatrogenic procedures, shifts in microbial flora, and potential acquisitions of new pathogens.

ORGANISMS OF INFECTION

Data from the University of Maryland Cancer Center (UMCC; formerly BCRC) as far back as 1969 and those of other cancer centers indicate that most infections are due to the organisms that have been colonizing at or near the site of infection [1,4,9,10,12,17,18]. Thus perirectal lesions are caused by gram-negative bacilli such as *Pseudomonas aeruginosa* and *Escherichia coli* present in the stool flora. Furthermore, there is a shift in the microbial flora of the upper aerodigestive tract toward a gram-negative enteric spectrum as the patient becomes ill and during the first few days of hospitalization. Any ill individual has major shifts in the organisms colonizing a specific area. For example, the oral flora changes from that composed primarily of aerobic and anaerobic gram-positive cocci and bacilli to an area that harbors many gram-negative bacilli. This change is related in part to changes in binding potential of the squamous epithelial cells lining the oral cavity. Studies by Johansen and co-workers [19] have shown that individuals who are hospitalized with illnesses of varying severity have an increased prevalence of gram-negative bacilli in the oropharynx. In addition, Valenti and others [20] have shown that the colonization with gram-negative organisms increases with the level of care and deteriorating clinical status. If a patient also receives broad spectrum antimicrobial therapy, colonizing flora will further shift toward either more resistant bacteria or to fungi such as *Candida* and *Torulopsis glabrata* [21,22]. The shift of the oropharyngeal flora toward the gram-negative organisms occurs even in the setting of reverse isolation [9], indicating that the patient's endogenous flora colonizing the lower intestinal tract promptly begins to colonize the upper aerodigestive tract. Furthermore, the acquisition of new organisms with colonization of both the upper aerodigestive and lower alimentary canal plays a major role in subsequent infection of the hospitalized patient. At the UMCC prior to the institution of strict infection prevention measures by the use of environmental control, half or more of all infections were caused by hospital-acquired organisms [10].

These concepts are of extreme importance because members of the health care delivery team must be fully cognizant of: (1) the spectrum of organisms that can colonize or be acquired by the patient receiving chemotherapy and (2) the propensity for these organisms to be of an enteric nature. Thus the concept of normal oral flora is not pertinent to these patients and any infection considered to originate in the upper aerodigestive tract as well as the lower respiratory tract must be considered to involve the gastrointestinal organisms as well as yeasts and gram-positive cocci.

SITES OF INFECTION

Virtually any site can be involved and nearly any organism can cause infection, particularly in the granulocytopenic patient. The majority of infections during neutropenia, however, occur in a limited number of sites with a relatively narrow spectrum of organisms (table 3–2). In a study by Schimpff and associates of the origin of infection in patients with acute nonlymphocytic leukemia, 75% of 111 infectious episodes in 48 patients occurred in five sites: the lower respiratory tract, the anorectum, skin and axilla, oropharynx, and urinary tract [10]. There has been a shift in the sites involved in infection with the introduction of effective prophylactic measures *(infra vide)* and the application of early appropriate broad spectrum antibiotics that cover the entire spectrum of gram-negative organisms such as *P. aeruginosa* as well as most other organisms. In comparison with the earlier data generated by Schimpff and co-workers, Ketchall and Rodriquez [23] in 1978 reported that the majority of infections occurred in the upper airway, the skin, and the urinary tract, in that order. In this report anorectal lesions fell to a lesser incidence and disseminated infections with unrecognized primary sites were the most frequent. More recently, oropharyngeal and periodontal infections have been recognized as a serious site of potential infection. In a recent report by Peterson and others, 24% of clinically documented infections in patients with acute nonlymphocytic leukemia at the UMCC were acute exacerbations of periodontal disease [24]. Thus with the evolution of appropriate prevention methods and appropriate systemic antibiotics both the organisms and the sites of infection constantly shift and the health care delivery team must be cognizant of all potential areas of involvement.

SIGNS AND SYMPTOMS OF INFECTION

The diagnosis of bacterial and fungal infections in the cancer patient is frequently difficult because of the impaired host defenses and concomitant granulocytopenia. In the presence of granulocytes, infection usually retains most of the signs and symptoms of infection such

Table 3–2. Sites of infection and spectrum of organisms

Lower respiratory tract
Enteric gram-negatives
Gram-positive cocci
Filamentous fungi
Yeasts
Upper aerodigestive tract (including mouth)
Enteric
Gram-positive cocci
Gram-negatives
Yeasts
Skin lesions
Gram-positive cocci
Diphtheroids
Enteric gram-negatives
Anal and perianal lesions
Enteric gram-negatives
Enterobacteriaceae
Urinary tract
Enteric gram-negatives
Enterobacteriaceae

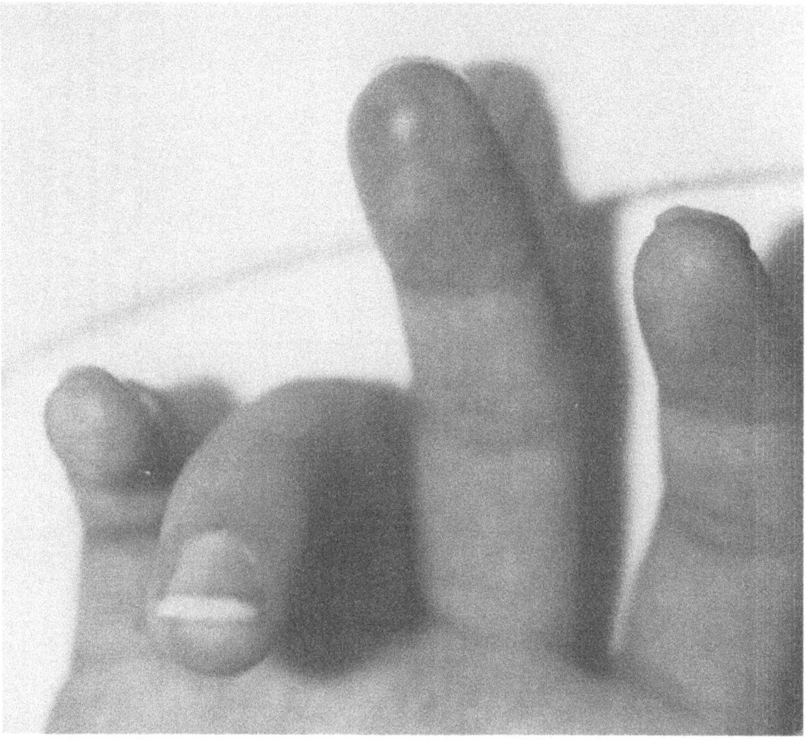

Figure 3–2. Third finger with mild erythema (note slightly darker colored area at the tip of this finger) and minimal tenderness following stick with crab shell. Despite the minimal findings, patient presented with temperature elevation of 101.6°F and multiple blood cultures growing *S. aureus.*

as pain, fever, swelling, erythema, and induration. In the absence of sufficient granulocytes, the inflammatory response is markedly impaired such that the usual signs and symptoms of infection may be lacking [25]. This is especially true for patients whose granulocyte counts are very low ($<100/\mu l$). The most reliable single sign of infection is the presence of fever $\geq$ 38°C (101.4°F). Another somewhat less reliable symptom is pain. For example, nearly all patients with infectious pharyngitis will have fever, some will have a sore throat, but only a small percentage will have an exudate or adenopathy. Likewise, patients with pneumonia may be febrile and occasionally have pulmonary signs such as rhonchi. Less often there is a sufficient inflammatory response to produce an infiltrate on chest x-ray; patients in this situation rarely produce sputum. Thus infection should be strongly suspected whenever a granulocytopenic patient is febrile or has a new painful lesion. Occasionally the findings suggesting infection are subtle (figure 3–2) or absent (figure 3–3). Despite the minimal findings, however, the patient may have a severe infection with bacteremia and may develop septic shock with a subsequent survival that can be measured in hours or days unless prompt appropriate therapeutic intervention is undertaken [26]. A careful physical examination with

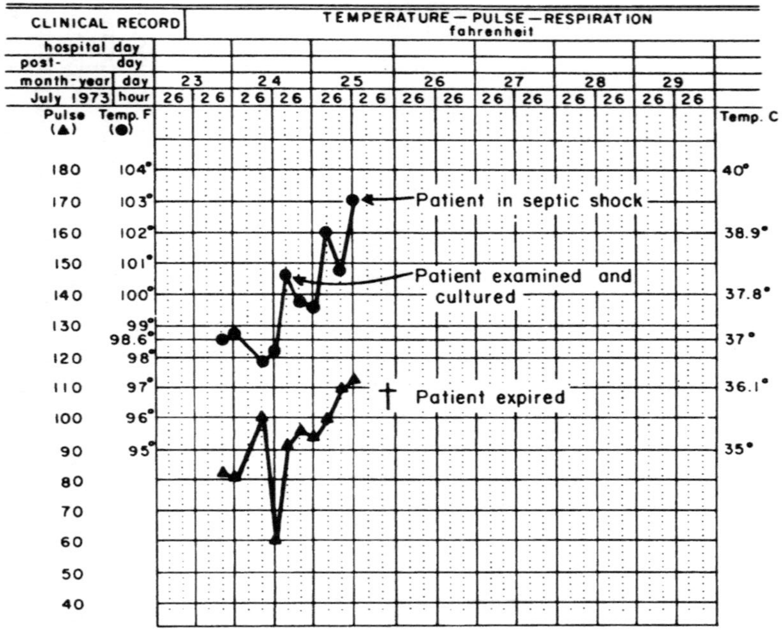

Figure 3–3. Clinical course of a febrile granulocytopenic patient with acute nonlymphocytic leukemia. Patient had completed induction chemotherapy with daunomycin and cytosine arabinoside resulting in profound granulocytopenia and transfusion dependence. Patient felt well until day illustrated when he developed a fever to 100.6°F following a platelet transfusion. History, physical examination, chest x-ray, and urinalysis were all negative. All cultures were taken (blood, urine, and surveillance cultures of nose, throat, and rectum) but antibiotics were withheld because the patient looked well and the fever was felt to be related to the platelet transfusion. Shortly thereafter the fever appeared to defervesce. However, six hours later the patient again had a febrile episode and shortly thereafter developed septic shock and died despite antibiotics and appropriate supportive measures. Blood cultures and rectal surveillance cultures drawn at the first and subsequent febrile episodes later grew *P. aeruginosa.* Source: Reproduced from Schimpff SC: Therapy of infection in patients with granulocytopenia, Med Clin North Am 61: 1101, 1977, reference 26 with permission W.B. Saunders.

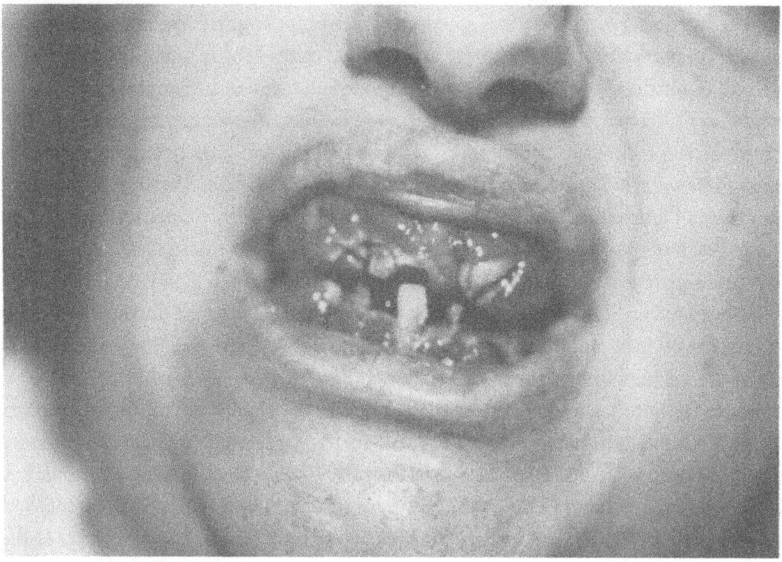

Figure 3–4. Patient with acute myelomonocytic leukemia showing leukemic infiltration of gums and gingiva. Despite the significant leukemic infiltration patient also has significant periodontitis which became manifest and a source of infection several days after initiation of induction chemotherapy. The infiltration receded due to the chemotherapy revealing the baseline periodontitis and patient eventually required multiple extractions.

special attention to the lungs, upper aerodigestive tract, perianal area, inguinal, and axillary areas must be combined with a careful history, urinalysis, and chest roentgenogram. Occasionally there may be difficulty distinguishing between underlying disease and concomitant infection (figure 3–4). The greater likelihood of an infectious episode and the severe consequence of delaying antimicrobial treatment dictate the use of appropriate therapeutic intervention. Thus all febrile episodes during granulocytopenia, unless known to be caused by other factors, must be considered as severe infections until proven otherwise.

EVALUATION OF INFECTION

Careful repeat history and physical examination, including the use of repeated diagnostic studies such as blood and urine cultures and chest roentgenography, will result in the vast majority of all febrile episodes being associated with clinically or microbiologically documented infections [26,27]. If all febrile episodes are divided into microbiologically documented infections, clinically documented infections (signs and symptoms of a specific site of infection), possible infections (equivocal signs and symptoms), and doubtful infections, it will be found that at least two thirds of the patients have microbiologically or clinically documented infections. If probable infections are included, approximately 80% of all febrile episodes are possibly or definitely infected; thus only a small percentage (approximately 20%) will have had a febrile episode unrelated to an infection [26,27].

Empiric antibiotic therapy

From the foregoing discussion it is apparent that prompt empiric institution of appropriate antibiotics is essential for the treatment and survival of the febrile granulocytopenic patient. A variety of antibiotic combinations will provide sufficient antimicrobial spectrum to treat the common infecting organisms [28]. The most frequently used combinations include two or three of the following antibiotics: synthetic or semisynthetic penicillin (with activity against *P. aeruginosa*), an aminoglycoside, and a cephalosporin. Various combinations of these classes of antibiotics have been tested in clinical trials of infection during granulocytopenia and each of the two or three drug combinations have been found to be highly efficacious using either parent drugs (cephalothin, carbenicillin, or gentamicin) or derivative (new generation) antibiotics [27–31]. Generally, greater than 70% of all documented infections will respond to such empiric antimicrobial therapy [28]. There are, however, some differences in the various antimicrobial therapies that need to be considered in general as well as specifically for both the organisms known to colonize the patient and the historical pattern of organisms for the individual institution. First, an aminoglycoside is generally inadequate as the only agent to provide antimicrobial activity for *P. aeruginosa* infection, especially in the granulocytopenic patient [27,28,30,32,33]. Second, it has been fairly well established that gram-negative infections, particularly gram-negative bacteremias, respond better to therapy if a synergistic combination of two antimicrobial agents is used [26,28,34]. Third, early trials with cephalothins plus any one of the aminoglycosides suggested an increased nephrotoxic potential for those two drug combinations, particularly in elderly individuals and those with some evidence of renal impairment [28,30,35,36]. Finally, the two-drug combination would best be chosen on the basis of surveillance cultures obtained from the host during or prior to periods of infection and the general experience with specific organisms at each institution [10,28]. This approach would take into consideration any unusual organism harbored or acquired by the patient or any special organism with an unusual susceptibility pattern known to recently cause infection at the given institution.

The primary determinant of response to a serious infection such as gram-negative bacteremia (provided the patient received at least one agent active against the organism) is whether or not there is a minimal return of marrow function as judged by increased marrow maturation or return of the peripheral granulocyte count [30,37–39]. An evaluation of such information at UMCC showed that 88% of patients with gram-negative bacteremia improved if they had some return of granulocytes, whereas only 22% of patients whose granulocyte count declined during therapy had such an improvement [37]. Thus although prompt antimicrobial therapy will provide response to most bacterial infections, serious infections such as gram-negative bacteremias can be an exception. When there is either a serious infection and no evidence of return of marrow function, or a decline in peripheral granulocytes and no evidence of improvement, the response rate is poor and such patients should be considered for granulocyte transfusions (37–39).

In the presence of a documented infection, the antibiotics are usually continued for a minimum of ten days or at least five days beyond the last febrile day [28]. There is, however, no unified opinion regarding the optimal time for discontinuation of therapy in the event that an infection cannot be documented. At some institutions, antibiotics, once started, are continued until the granulocyte count returns. Evidence from UMCC and other institu-

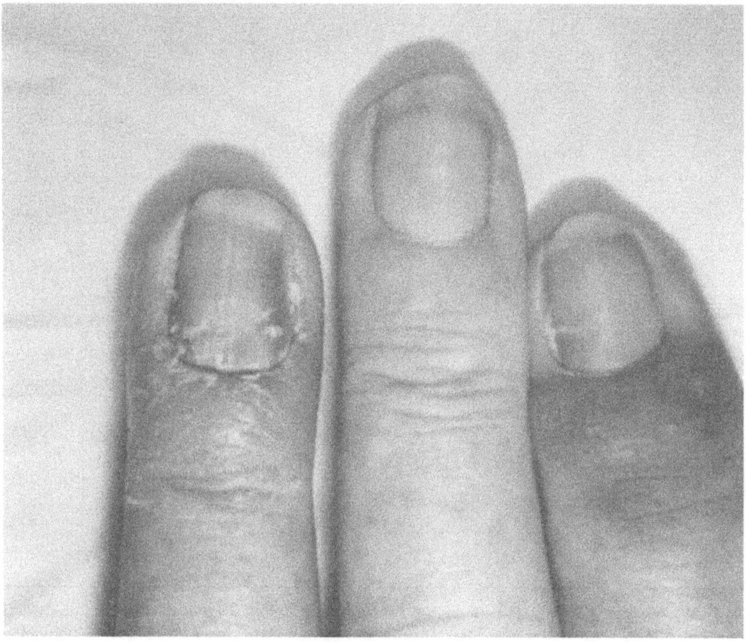

Figure 3–5. Mild paronychia on finger in patient with acute leukemia. Patient developed fever and chills while on antibiotics and scrapings from finger grew *C. albicans* on culture. Blood cultures also grew *C. albicans,* indicating the propensity for dissemination of infection.

tions suggests that the incidence of subsequent bacterial and fungal infections increases with the time of antibiotic exposure [22,28,30]. There would thus appear to be some reason for the discontinuation of antibiotics in the absence of a documented infection. Our practice at UMCC is to discontinue antibiotics after approximately four days if a complete and thorough history and physical examination and laboratory evaluation are nonrevealing and the patient appears stable and nontoxic. For any given patient, however, the decision should be based upon careful repeated evaluations with close follow-up so that antimicrobial therapy can be reinstituted if warranted.

With the increased use of broad spectrum antibacterial agents and improved survival from bacterial infections, there has been an increasing number of fungal infections with organisms such as *Aspergillus spp., Candida spp.,* and others [22,28,40,41]. There is convincing evidence that successful treatment of invasive systemic mycoses is associated with early diagnosis and prompt institution of antifungal agents such as amphotericin-B [28,42,43]. In many instances the diagnosis requires an aggressive approach including bronchial biopsies, bronchial brushings, transbronchial biopsies, percutaneous lung biopsies, or open lung biopsies for pulmonary infiltrates. As in the situation with bacterial diseases, the fungal diseases may have an insidious onset, with minimal lesions arising either in the mouth or other areas (figure 3–5). Without proper antifungal treatment, progressive invasive disease

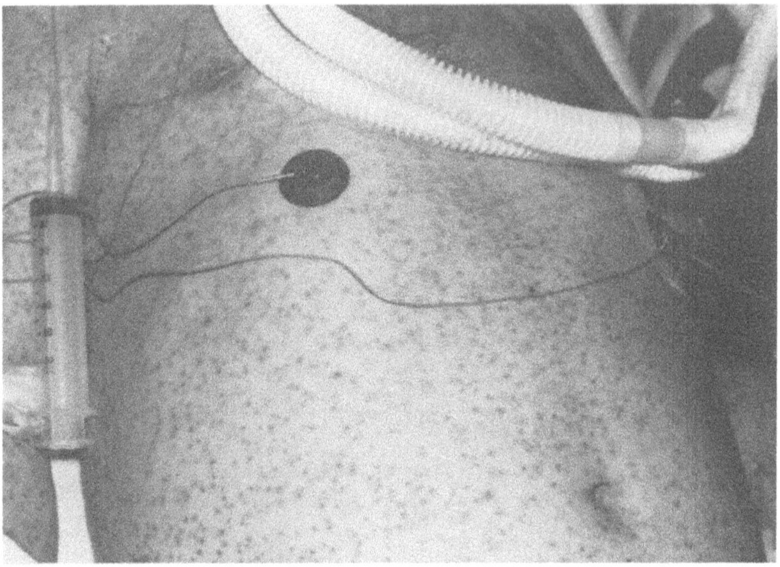

Figure 3–6. Disseminated candidiasis in patient with acute leukemia. Patient developed oral candidiasis with dysphagia. Smears showed typical hyphal forms and cultures later grew *C. albicans.* Fever and chills were associated with a few red punctate lesions suggestive of echthyma gangrenosa. This prompted further antibacterial antibiotics. Within 48 hours of the first skin lesions, patient demonstrated widespread dissemination as seen here with blood cultures growing *C. albicans.*

with systemic dissemination can result (figure 3–6). Furthermore, delay in therapy of such diseases as aspergillosis will allow the natural progression of arterial invasion, distal infarction, and subsequent invasion of the necrotic tissue by the fungus such that antibiotics will penetrate poorly and patient response will be minimal [44]. Similar to the bacterial organisms, the invasive mycoses can frequently be predicted on the basis of surveillance cultures; there is evidence to suggest that *T. glabrata, Candida spp.,* and *Aspergillus flavus* have been associated with local colonization and tissue invasion following systemic broad spectrum antibacterial antibiotics [22,41,44].

The antifungal drugs currently available include amphotericin-B, 5-fluorocytosine (5-FC), and the imidazoles, miconazole, and ketoconazole. The two imidazoles have antifungal properties in vitro [45]. However, there is very little information from clinical trials in neutropenic patients [46]. There are also reports that suggest a lack of efficacy [47] or an adverse effect in animal models [48]. These two imidazoles have thus not been satisfactorily established as clinically effective for invasive fungal infections in the granulocytopenic patient. The role of these agents as fungal prophylaxis is currently being explored. 5-FC has been reported to have activity in the treatment of patients with systemic mycoses, especially yeast such as *Candida spp.* and *T. glabrata.* Its efficacy in the neutropenic patient has not been adequately established and resistance in many species has been noted [49]. Amphotericin-B has been shown to be effective in a variety of systemic mycoses, including disseminated mycoses in the granulocytopenic patient [42,50]. This drug therefore remains the drug of choice for the systemic mycoses, although it has significant morbidity including frequent induction of renal impairment [50]. Thus empiric therapy for suspected fungal infections still remains to be established because: (1) there is little enthusiasm for the use of amphotericin-B because of its morbidity; and (2) although preliminary data suggest possible activity, there is still insufficient data for the use of the imidazoles or 5-FC as empiric therapy. There is laboratory and animal model data that suggest that amphotericin-B plus either rifampin or 5-FC will act synergistically against the fungi that tend to infect the granulocytopenic patient [51,52]. Thus it is conceivable that one of the combinations may prove better than amphotericin-B alone. Currently at our center, any patient who develops a new febrile episode while granulocytopenic and who has received broad spectrum antibiotic therapy is considered for possible empiric antifungal therapy. The decision is usually made on the basis of invasive tests appropriate to the site of infection (e.g., esophagoscopy for esophagitis, bronchoscopy with bronchial brushing for pulmonary infection, and so on). If, however, patients cannot tolerate the invasive procedure (e.g., in the setting of uncorrectable bleeding parameters), the choice of therapy may rest primarily upon consideration of the predisposing factors and can be based on epidemiologic factors, such as colonization, or presence of filamentous fungi on nose cultures [53].

INFECTION PREVENTION

One major means to reduce the incidence of infection in the cancer patient is to develop and follow infection prevention techniques [12,18]. These would include, wherever possible, the avoidance of invasive and manipulative techniques, avoidance of indwelling catheters, reduction in the acquisition of exogenous organisms, and the suppression of potentially pathogenic host organisms. Since manipulative techniques such as endoscopy or those as simple as scaling the teeth (as prophylaxis) cannot uniformly be avoided, this would suggest that procedure-associated bacteremias might be anticipated. Thus prophylactic systemic antibiotics with appropriate antimicrobial spectrum to cover the manipulative technique would be worthwhile. At our center, patients who are to undergo such manipulative techniques and are not otherwise febrile or felt to be infected are given either 24 to 48 hours of coverage with antibiotics appropriate to the organisms found on surveillance cultures in that site or given sufficient broad spectrum activity to provide antimicrobial coverage for all microorganisms that may have shifted to the site that is to be manipulated.

Indwelling urinary catheters are utilized only in the setting of septic shock and incontinence. Similarly, indwelling intravenous catheters are avoided except as indicated for shock, central venous pressure monitoring, and so on. Peripheral venous access at our center is accomplished by changing butterfly needles every 48 hours. Recent experience with long-term indwelling (Hickman) venous catheters has shown that this specially designed catheter of silicone rubber, which utilizes separate skin entrance and cuffed exit sites, can be maintained for prolonged periods of time with careful attention to details of aseptic technique for changing dressings and routine care [54].

Another major area in which the incidence of infection might be reduced would be to decrease the acquisition of exogenous organisms [12,18]. It has been shown by our group

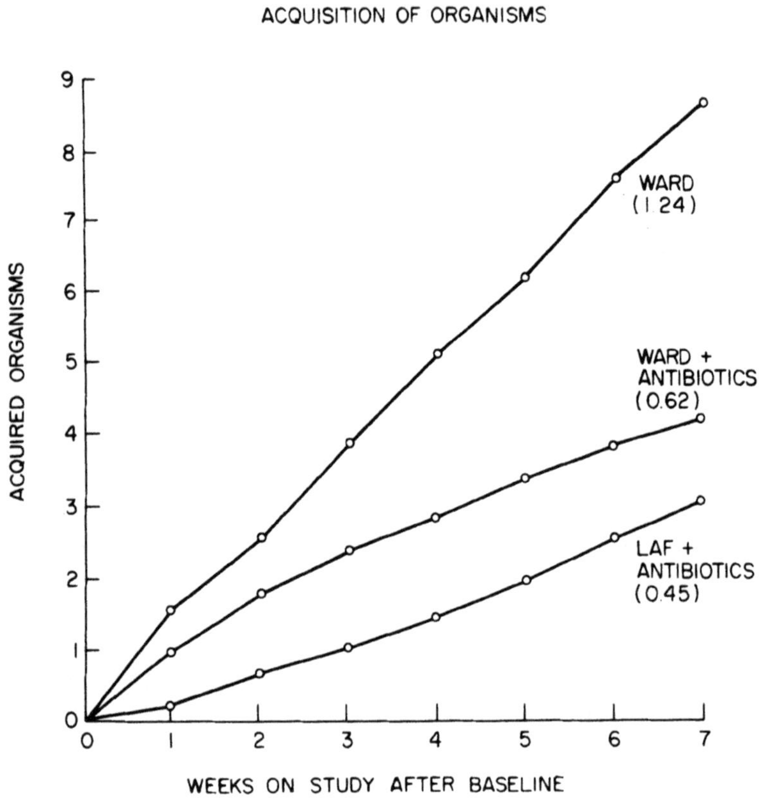

Figure 3–7. Incidence of acquisition of potentially pathogenic organisms over time during initial treatment for acute leukemia. Patients without preventive measures (ward alone) had the greatest rate of acquisition while those patients receiving full preventive measures of reverse isolation and air filtration and nonabsorbable antibiotics had the lowest acquisition. (Source: Reproduced from Schimpff SC: Infection prevention in patients with cancer and granulocytopenia. In Greico (ed), *Infections in the Abnormal Host* with permission by Yorke Medical Books)

and others [55,56] that patients maintained in the hospital setting, who neither practice nor receive specific techniques at reduction in organisms acquisition, will have a constant rate of new organism acquisition with time (figure 3–7). This acquisition can come from food, as well as contact with the ubiquitous gram-negative organisms present in soil, water, plants, and from hands and equipment of hospital personnel. Thus the utilization of cooked foods and the avoidance of fresh foods such as mixed salads, will eliminate a major source of new organism acquisition [12,18]. The avoidance of fresh flowers or cut flowers in water in the patient's room will also reduce the opportunity for access to waterborne gram-negative bacteria such as *P. aeruginosa* [57].

The skin, especially the hands, has long been known to be a source of microorganisms, as are many instruments that are utilized in common between patients, such as stethoscopes, blood pressure cuffs, and even invasive instruments such as endoscopes [12,13,14]. Thus careful attention to hand washing and the cleansing of instrumentation can be a major method for the reduction in new organism acquisition. Splash from sink drains may also contain a variety of gram-negative organisms [12], and careful attention to cleaning of these areas is necessary to decrease this source of organism acquisition. Airborne organisms can be aerosolized from patient and staff expectorations (coughing) as well as a variety of other sources such as the flushing of toilets, the shaking of dirty linens, and air conditioners. The only effective way to eliminate the airborne contamination is to utilize barrier isolation with laminar air flow high efficiency, particulate air filtration systems [9,18,55,56]. The use of these specially designed rooms along with alimentary canal flora suppression is known to reduce the acquisition of new organisms and to decrease infectious morbidity. It needs further evaluation for its cost-effectiveness as well as its ability to improve the remission rate in patients with acute leukemia and other marrow failure states. The use of standard reverse isolation is illogical despite its use for years as infection prevention. Most single-room reverse-isolation procedures do not interfere with the major routes of acquisition or the potential pathogens that cause infection. Little or no attention is paid to the supplies in the room, the food, or the water which are the most common sources of new organism acquisition. Furthermore, the acquisition of hospital organisms is probably more likely to be by resistant flora. Thus the patient with granulocytopenia who is not febrile and can be easily brought back and forth to the clinic facility can frequently fare well at home under self-care.

Another productive avenue for infection prevention is the use of antimicrobial agents in the suppression of host digestive tract flora. One approach has been to use oral nonabsorbable agents such as nystatin, vancomycin, and gentamicin [9,55]. This technique combined with a cooked food diet is highly effective in maintaining both low colony counts of organisms recoverable from the anus or stool (figure 3–7) and reduced counts of organisms from the oral cavity [9,18,55,58]. The difficulty with this procedure is the high cost of daily administration, the unpleasant taste leading to poor compliance, the rapid recolonization (often with undesirable organisms) in the absence of good compliance, and the possibility of inducing gentamicin-resistant organisms [12,18,59].

Another technique in which only the aerobic flora are suppressed has been developed using trimethoprim/sulfamethoxazol and similar agents [60–64]. These permit the anaerobic flora to remain which in turn impart colonization resistance for other organisms [60,63]. With this technique 10^4 more organisms are needed to induce colonization than in the situation of total suppression with poor compliance [63]. This method is also far less expensive, more convenient in dose frequency, and has been shown effective in several tumor types such as acute leukemia and small-cell carcinoma of the lung [61–64]. Further studies with this method are, however, still needed to assess its impact on response, duration of myeloid suppression, and emergence of resistant organisms.

PATIENT'S ROLE

The patient as well as the health care staff needs appropriate background to reduce the incidence of infection. Most adults have some periodontal disease that can serve as a nidus of infection during periods of chemotherapy-induced myelosuppression [24]. An aggressive approach of good dental hygiene, including brushing and flossing under careful supervision, appears necessary to reduce the incidence of infection within the oral cavity. In addition, adequate patient education is critically important since matters of personal hygiene, including proper bathing techniques, oral hygiene, hand washing, and the cleansing of the axilla and the inguinal areas with antiseptic agents, all help reduce the number of potentially pathogenic organisms. The patient should also be instructed to act as the monitor of staff and visitor behavior so that no one is allowed to sit on the bed, perform examinations, draw blood, and so on without first washing hands, or bring gifts such as cut flowers. Furthermore, the patient should be directed not to get out of bed without using slippers or to place feet or other external objects upon the bed where he or she will lie. Finally, the knowledge and recognition by the patient of the personal changes that may indicate infection, such as fever or areas of pain, would allow the patient to notify the nurse or physician at the earliest possible time so that early appropriate intervention may be undertaken. With these measures both infection prevention and early empiric therapy are best instituted for the patient's benefit.

SUMMARY

Although infection prevention techniques are presently used extensively for many cancer patients, infections can occur frequently in those patients. This problem is particularly severe in patients who are receiving myelosuppressive or immunosuppressive treatment. Care of the infected cancer patient is complex, requiring thorough knowledge by and cooperation among the health team. The team must be aware of factors that can lead to infections, as well as sites, signs and symptoms, treatment and, ideally, prevention of such complications. Through a comprehensive approach to these patients, their risk from infection can be minimized.

REFERENCES

1. Remington JS, Schimpff SC, Hughes WT, et al: Life-threatening infections in the compromised host. In *Current Chemotherapy: Proceedings of the 10th International Congress of Chemotherapy,* Washington, D.C., American Society for Microbiology, 1978, pp. 37–42.
2. Aisner J, Schiffer CA, Wiernik PH: Cell support. In *Fundamentals of Clinical Hematology,* Spivak S (ed), Hagerstown, Md, Harper & Row, 1980, pp 357–368.
3. Pennington JE: Fever, neutropenia and malignancy: A clinical syndrome in evolution. Cancer 39: 1345–1349, 1977.
4. Levine AS, Schimpff SC, Graw RG Jr, et al.: Hematologic malignancies and other marrow failure states: progress in the management of complicating infections. Sem. Hematol 11: 141–201, 1974.
5. Bodey GP: Microbiologic aspects in patients with acute leukemia. Hum Pathol 5: 687–698, 1974.
6. Winston DJ, Gale RP, Meyer DV, et al.: Infectious complications of human bone marrow transplantation. Medicine (Baltimore) 58: 1–31, 1979.
7. Stinson EB, Bieber CP, Griepp RB, et al.: Infectious complications after cardiac transplantation in man. Ann Intern Med 74: 22–36, 1971.
8. Bodey GP, Buckley M, Sathe YS, et al.: Quantitative relationships between circulating leukocytes and infection in patients with acute leukemia. Ann Intern Med 64: 328–340, 1966.
9. Schimpff SC, Hahn DM, Brouillet MD, et al.: Infection prevention in acute leukemia: comparison of basic infection prevention techniques, with standard room reverse isolation or with reverse isolation and added air filtration. Leuk Res 2: 231–240, 1978.
10. Schimpff SC, Young VM, Greene WH, et al.: Origin of infection in acute nonlymphocytic leukemia: significance of hospital acquisition of potential pathogens. Ann Intern Med 77: 707–714, 1972.
11. Remington JS: The compromised host. Hosp Pract 7: 59–70, 1972.

12. Schimpff SC, Young VM: Epidemiology and prevention of infection in the compromised host. In *Clinical Approach to Infection in the Compromised Host,* Rubin RH and Young LS (eds), New York, Plenum Publishing, 1981, pp 5–33.
13. Greene WH, Moody M, Hartley R, et al.: Esophagoscopy as a source of *Pseudomonas aeruginosa* sepsis in patients with acute leukemia: the need for sterilization of endoscopes. Gastroenterology 67: 912–919, 1974.
14. LeFrock JL, Ellis CA, Turchik JB, et al.: Transient bacteremia associated with sigmoidoscopy. N Engl J Med 289: 467–469, 1973.
15. Felix JE, Rosen S, App GR: Detection of bacteremia after the use of an oral irrigation device in subjects with periodontitis. J Periodontol 42: 785–787, 1971.
16. Hahn DM, Schimpff SC, Fortner CL, et al.: Infection in acute leukemia patients receiving oral non-absorbable antibiotics. Antimicrob Agents Chemother 13: 958–964, 1978.
17. Schimpff SC, Moody M, Young VM: Relationship of colonization with *Pseudomonas aeruginosa* to development of *Pseudomonas* bacteremia in cancer patients. Antimicrob Agents Chemother 10: 240–244, 1970.
18. Schimpff SC: Infection prevention in patients with cancer and granulocytopenia. In *Infections in the Abnormal Host,* MH Greco (ed), New York, Yorke Medical Books, 1980, pp 926–950.
19. Johanson WG, Pierce AK, Sanford JP: Changing pharvngeal bacterial flora of hospitalized patients: emergence of gram-negative bacilli. N Engl J Med 281: 1137–1140, 1969.
20. Valenti WM, Trudell RG, Bentley DW: Factors predisposing to oropharyngeal colonization with gram-negative bacilli in the aged. N Engl J Med 298: 1108–1111, 1978.
21. Spencer RC, Philip JR: Effect of previous antimicrobial therapy on bacteriological findings in patients with primary pneumonia. Lancet 2: 349–350, 1973.
22. Aisner J, Schimpff SC, Hahn DM, et al.: Fungal infections in patients with cancer: changing frequency associated with broad spectrum antibiotics. Clin Res 23: 586A, 1976.
23. Ketchel SJ, Rodriquez V: Acute infections in cancer patients. Semin Oncol 5: 167–179, 1978.
24. Peterson D, Overholser CD, Newman KA, et al.: Periodontal infection in patients (pts) with acute nonlymphocytic leukemia (ANLL). Proc Am Soc Clin Oncol 20: 351, 1979.
25. Sickles EA, Greene WH, Wiernik PH: Clinical presentation of infection in granulocytopenic patients. Arch Intern Med 135: 715–719, 1975.
26. Schimpff SC: Therapy of infections in patients with granulocytopenia. Med Clin North Am 61: 1101–1118, 1972.
27. Schimpff SC, Satterlee W, Young VM, et al.: Empiric therapy with carbenicillin and gentamicin for febrile patients with cancer and granulocytopenia. N Engl J Med 284: 1061–1065, 1971.
28. Schimpff SC, Aisner J: Commentary: empiric antibiotic therapy. Cancer Treat Rep 62: 673–680, 1978.
29. Schimpff SC, Landesman D, Hahn DM, et al.: Ticarcillin in combination with cephalothin or gentamicin as empiric antibiotic therapy in granulocytopenic cancer patients. Antimicrob Agents Chemother 10: 837–844, 1976.
30. EORTC Antimicrobial Therapy Project Group: Three antibiotic regimens in the treatment of infection in febrile granulocytopenic patients with cancer. J Infect Dis 137: 14–29, 1978.
31. DeJongh CA, Wade JC, Schimpff SC, et al.: Empiric antibiotic therapy for suspected infection in granulocytopenic cancer patients: a comparison between the combination of moxalactam plus amikacin and ticarcillin plus amikacin. Am J Med 73: 89–96, 1982.
32. Bodey GP, Middleman E, Umsawadi T, et al.: Infections in cancer patients: results with gentamicin sulfate therapy. Cancer 29: 1697–1701, 1972.
33. Dale DC, Reynolds HY, Pennington JE, et al.: Granulocyte transfusion therapy of experimental *Pseudomonas* pneumonia. J Clin Invest 54: 664–671, 1974.
34. Klastersky J, Munier-Charpentier F, Prevost JM: Significance of antimicrobial synergism for the outcome of gram-negative sepsis. Am J Med Sci 273: 157–167, 1977.
35. Wade JC, Smith CR, Petty BG, et al.: Cephalothin plus an aminoglycoside is more nephrotoxic than methicillin plus an aminoglycoside. Lancet 2: 604–606, 1978.
36. Wade JC, Schimpff SC, Wiernik PH: Antibiotic combination-associated nephrotoxicity in granulocytopenic patients with cancer. Arch Intern Med 141: 1789–1793, 1982.
37. Love LJ, Schimpff SC, Schiffer CA, et al.: Improved prognosis for granulocytopenic patients with gram-negative bacteremia. Am J Med 68: 643–646, 1980.
38. Herzig RH, Herzig GP, Graw RG Jr, et al.: Granulocyte transfusion therapy for gram-negative septicemia. N Engl J Med 296: 701–705, 1977.
39. Aisner J, Schiffer CA, Wiernik PH: Granulocyte transfusion: evaluation of factors influencing results and a comparison of filtration and intermittent centrifugation leukopheresis. Br J Haematol 38: 121–129, 1978.

40. Krick JA, Remington JS: Opportunistic invasion fungal infections in patients with leukemia and lymphoma. Clin Haematol 5: 149–310, 1976.
41. Aisner J, Schimpff SC, Sutherland JC, et al.: *Torulopsis glabrata* infections in patients with cancer: increasing incidence and relationship to colonization. Am J Med 61: 23–28, 1976.
42. Aisner J, Schimpff SC, Wiernik PH: Treatment of invasive aspergillosis: relation of early diagnosis and treatment to response. Ann Intern Med 86: 539–543, 1977.
43. Pennington JE: Aspergillus lung disease. Med Clin North Am 64: 475–490, 1980.
44. Aisner J, Schimpff SC: Aspergillosis. In *Clinical Medicine,* Spittell JA Jr (ed), Philadelphia, Harper & Row, 1981, pp 1–14.
45. Dixon D, Shadomy S, Shadomy HJ, et al.: Comparison of the *in vitro* antifungal activities of miconazole and a new imidazole R41400. J Infect Dis 138: 245–248, 1978.
46. Jordan WM, Brodey GP, Rodriguez V, et al.: Miconazole therapy for treatment of fungal infections in cancer patients. Antimicrob Agents Chemother 16: 792–797, 1979.
47. Feinstein V, Elting L, Bodey GP: Treatment of antibiotic resistant fever with trimethoprim-sulfamethoxazole ± miconazole in cancer patients. Proc 21st Interscience Conference on Antimicrobial Agents and Chemotherapy, Abst 797, Washington, D.C., American Society Microbiology, 1981.
48. Bader-Hawley L: Treatment of invasive aspergillosis in immunocompromised mice with high dose ketoconazole. Proc 21st Interscience Conference on Antimicrobial Agents and Chemotherapy, Abst 277, Washington, D.C., American Society Microbiology, 1981.
49. Bennett SE: Drugs 5 years later: fluorocytosine. Ann Intern Med 86: 319–322, 1977.
50. Bennett VE: Chemotherapy of the systemic mycoses. N Engl J Med 290: 320–323, 1974.
51. Kitahara M, Seth VK, Medoff G, et al.: Activity of amphotericin-B, 5-fluorocytosine and rifampin against 6 clinical isolates of *Aspergillus.* Antimicrob Agents Chemother 9: 915–919, 1976.
52. Moody MR, Young VM, Morris MJ, et al.: *In vitro* activities of miconazole, miconazole nitrate, and ketoconazole alone and combined with rifampin against *Candida spp* and *Torulopsis glabrata* recovered from patient with cancer. Antimicrob Agents Chemother 17: 571–875, 1980.
53. Aisner J, Murillo J, Schimpff SC, et al.: Invasive aspergillosis in acute leukemia: correlation with nose cultures and antibiotic use. Ann Intern Med 90: 4–9, 1979.
54. Wade JC, Newman KA, Schimpff SC, et al.: Two methods for improved venous access in acute leukemia patients. JAMA 246: 140–144, 1981.
55. Schimpff SC, Greene WH, Young VM, et al.: Infection prevention in acute nonlymphocytic leukemia: laminar air flow room reverse isolation with oral, nonabsorbable antibiotic prophylaxis. Ann Intern Med 82: 351–358, 1975.
56. Dietrich M, Gaus W, Vossen J, et al.: Prospective isolation and antimicrobial decontamination in patients with high susceptibility to infection: a prospective cooperative group study of gnotobiotic care in acute leukemia patients. Clin Res Infect 5: 3–10, 1977.
57. Taplin D, Mertz PM: Flower vases in hospitals as reservoirs of pathogens. Lancet 2: 1279–1281, 1973.
58. Schimpff SC: Protected environments for the treatment of high risk cancer patients. In *Controversies in Oncology,* PH Wiernik (ed), New York, John Wiley & Sons, 1982, pp 247–265.
59. Hahn DM, Schimpff SC, Fortner CL, et al.: Infection in acute leukemia patients receiving non-absorbable antibiotics. Antimicrob Agents Chemother 13: 958–964, 1978.
60. van der Waaij D: The colonization resistance of the digestive tract in experimental animals and its consequences for infection prevention, acquisition of new bacteria and the prevention of spread of bacteria between cage mates. In *New Criteria for Antimicrobial Therapy: Maintenance of Digestive Tract Colonization Resistance,* van der Waaij D, Verhoef J (eds), Excerpta Medica Amsterdam, 1979, pp 43–53.
61. Gurwith MJ, Brunton JL, Bank LA, et al.: A prospective controlled investigation of prophylactic trimethoprim/sulfamethoxazole in hospitalized granulocytopenic patients. Am J Med 66: 248–255, 1979.
62. Wade JC, Schimpff SC, Hargadon MT, et al.: A comparison of trimethoprim-sulfamethoxazole plus nystatin with gentamicin plus nystatin in the prevention of infections in acute leukemia. N Engl J Med 304: 1057–1062, 1981.
63. Hargadon MT, Young VM, Schimpff SC, et al.: Selective suppression of alimentary tract microbial flora as prophylaxis during granulocytopenia. Antimicrob Agents Chemother 20: 620–624, 1981.
64. deJongh CA, Wade J, Finley R, et al.: Double blind randomized comparison of trimethoprim/sulfamethoxazole versus placebo for prophylaxis of infection in patients with oat cell carcinoma. Proc Am Soc Clin Oncol 1: 55, 1982.

4. ORAL MICROBIAL CHANGES AND INFECTIONS DURING CANCER CHEMOTHERAPY

SAMUEL DREIZEN, D.D.S., M.D.
LEE R. BROWN, Ph. D.

RATIONALE FOR CANCER CHEMOTHERAPY

The modern history of cancer chemotherapy began during World War II with the demonstration that several nitrogen mustard compounds acting as alkylating agents were effective in the treatment of Hodgkin's disease, malignant lymphoma, chronic leukemias, and allied disorders [1]. In the intervening years, there has been a striking increase in the number of clinically active anticancer chemicals and in the types of malignant disease that have been found to be drug responsive. Today, the antineoplastic drugs are used as primary treatment for many widely disseminated cancers and as adjunctive treatment to surgery and radiotherapy for reduction of tumor bulk, eradication of localized malignancies, and destruction of malignant cells that escape surgical resection or exposure to ionizing radiation. Cancers most amenable to cure or control by the presently available chemotherapeutic agents are listed in table 4–1 [2].

All antineoplastic drugs kill or impair susceptible tumor cells by blocking a drug-sensitive biochemical or metabolic pathway. Some, like the cell-cycle-specific antimetabolites, act by inhibiting DNA synthesis and are most effective against rapidly dividing cells. Others, like the alkylating agents, act by interfering with DNA, RNA, and protein synthesis and are thus effective against both proliferating and resting cells. All are extremely potent and have only a slight margin of safety between the tumoricidal and toxic dose.

TYPES OF CANCER CHEMOTHERAPY

Antitumor drugs cannot distinguish between cancer cells and normal cells and are thus potentially damaging to both. The primary objective of cancer chemotherapy is to maxi-

D.E. Peterson and S.T. Sonis (eds.), ORAL COMPLICATIONS OF CANCER CHEMOTHERAPY, 41-77.

Table 4–1. Cancers curable or controllable by chemotherapy

Curable (Long-Term Survival)	Controllable (Improved-Survival)
Acute leukemia in children	Acute leukemia in adults
Burkitt's lymphoma	Adrenal cortical carcinoma
Choriocarcinoma	Breast carcinoma
Embryonal rhabdomyosarcoma	Endometrial carcinoma
Ewing's sarcoma	Lymphocytic lymphoma
Hodgkin's disease	Malignant insulinoma
Retinoblastoma	Neuroblastoma
Skin cancer	Osteogenic sarcoma
Testicular carcinoma	Ovarian carcinoma
Wilms' tumor	Prostatic carcinoma

mize the destruction of cancer cells and to minimize the damage to normal cells. Combining drugs with different mechanisms of action and with different sites of toxicity diminishes the risk of injury to normal cells by lowering the effective dose of each component. The effectiveness of phase-specific drugs depends upon a repeating schedule or infusion, whereas cycle-specific drugs are most effective in large single doses. Combination cancer chemotherapy is thus usually given as a series of intermittent courses rather than by long-term continuous administration. Intermittent chemotherapy allows time for recovery and restoration of tissues unintentionally and unavoidably compromised by the drugs, thereby lessening the possibility of fatal consequences.

IMMUNOSUPPRESSIVE ACTION OF CANCER CHEMOTHERAPY

Both the bone marrow and the oral mucosal epithelium are endowed with rates of cell replication comparable to those of fast-growing tumors. Consequently, these structures are particularly vulnerable to the depressant action of the tumoricidal chemicals. Drug-induced ablation of the stem cells that mature into granulocytes and lymphocytes markedly reduces the protection afforded by the immune process [3]. Specifically, antigen uptake or processing is impaired by actinomycin D, corticosteroids, and cyclophosphamide; antigen recognition or precursor cell destruction is interfered with by corticosteroids and cyclophosphamide; lymphoblastoid blastogenesis is inhibited by actinomycin D, cyclophosphamide, L-asparaginase, 5-fluorouracil, and 6-mercaptopurine; lymphoblastoid proliferation is diminished by actinomycin D, cytosine arabinoside, methotrexate, and vinca alkaloids; antibody production is prevented by cyclophosphamide and the effector reactions of cell-mediated and humoral immunity are suppressed by corticosteroids. Antitumor agents also interfere with the inflammatory response wherein neutrophils initially migrate to the site of inflammation followed by mononuclear cells. Among the most suppressive of this response are procarbazine, methotrexate, 6-mercaptopurine, actinomycin D, cyclophosphamide, and corticosteroids. The cumulative effect is immunosuppression characterized by depression of phagocytic activity, abolition of antibody production, inhibition of the development of delayed hypersensitivity, and blocking of the mononuclear phase of the inflammatory reaction. Immunosuppression thus renders the host exceedingly vulnerable to bacterial, fungal, viral, and mixed infections.

The extent of immunosuppression varies with the drug and duration of administration. Recovery of immune responsiveness after a single dose of a cytostatic agent usually takes 48 to 72 hours. When multiple drug protocols are used, the recovery period is prolonged. Several weeks may be required for restitution of immunocompetence after two to three years of combination chemotherapy [4].

MYELOSUPPRESSIVE ACTION OF CANCER CHEMOTHERAPY

The greater the degree and duration of neutropenia and lymphocytopenia, the greater the liability to infection. Patients with granulocyte or lymphocyte counts of less than $100/mm^3$ in the peripheral blood have a greater than 50% chance of developing an infection somewhere in the body [3]. Persistence of this level for three weeks increases the risk to 100% [5]. The most severe infections are more commonly associated with neutropenia than with lymphocytopenia, since chemotherapeutic agents often have a more profound effect on the concentration of circulating neutrophils than on circulating lymphocytes. Among the most frequent sites of infection in the immunoincompetent patient are the mouth and oropharynx.

Phagocytic activity is a function of the maturational state of the granulocyte. Immature cells such as the myeloblast do not have any phagocytic activity. Progranulocytes are the first cells in the series to show slight phagocytic action. There follows a great increase in phagocytosis as the cells mature through the metamyelocyte, band-cell, and polymorphonuclear-cell stages. In contrast, cells of the lymphoid series from lymphoblast to lymphocyte do not have any phagocytic potential [6]. Patients may also have adequate numbers of circulating neutrophils and still be susceptible to infection due to impaired neutrophil function secondary to the disease or to the therapy.

CYTOTOXIC ACTION OF CANCER CHEMOTHERAPY

Many of the drugs used in the treatment of cancer are cytotoxic to the oral mucosa, impeding replication, growth, and maturation of the epithelial cells [7,8]. This effect is expressed clinically by thinning, denudation, and ulceration of the surface mucosa. The mucosal atrophy has been attributed to drug-suppressed proliferation of the basal-cell layer [9]. Although the oral reactions to the stomatotoxic anticancer drugs are, in general, dose-related, patients differ substantially in their capacity to tolerate a given dose of a cytotoxic drug or combination of drugs. There is considerably more interpatient than intrapatient variation in this regard. Those who develop oral manifestations during the initial course of treatment will almost certainly develop similar lesions during each subsequent course unless the drugs are changed or the dosage is lowered.

Drug-induced oral mucositis usually begins with burning and reddening of the mucosa within the first 24 hours after the start of administration, although some drugs have a delayed action. The premonitory stage is followed in one to three days by the emergence of excrutiatingly painful denudations and erosions that continue to intensify as long as the drug is given. The mucositis usually lasts for one to two weeks after treatment is discontinued. It is often magnified by the trauma-intense mouth environment. No other part of the body is as routinely and repeatedly exposed to as much chemical, physical, thermal, microbial, and mechanical trauma as the mouth. The drug-induced and trauma-intensified reduction in tissue barriers to infection and the drug-precipitated myelosuppression and immunosuppression combine to make the mouth a favorite target site for infection in patients undergoing cancer chemotherapy. Every such infection, regardless of cause, is potentially lethal since the damaged mucosa may serve as a portal of entry to the bloodstream, leading to fulminating septicemia and widespread hematogenous dissemination.

CANCER CHEMOTHERAPY-INDUCED ORAL INFECTIONS

The vast majority of oral infections in hospitalized patients receiving cancer chemotherapy are opportunistic or nosocomial in nature. They stem from exposure of the drug and disease-debilitated patient to the hospital population and environment. Both endogenous and exogenous microorganisms are capable of producing life-threatening oral infections in patients with reduced host defenses. Exogenous organisms acquired in the hospital are frequently more virulent and more resistant to antibiotics than are the endogenous microflora. Prime sources of the exogenous gram-negative aerobic bacilli are the hospital food, water, plumbing, and bathroom facilities; of exogenous *Staphylococcus aureus,* the hospital personnel; of exogenous *Aspergillus spp.,* the hospital air [10].

Microbiologic surveillance studies of patients treated for acute nonlymphocytic leukemia starting on admission and continuing until death or discharge have shown that all such patients acquire multiple potential pathogens while in hospital [11]. Whereas most of the documented infections arose from the patients' endogenous microflora, many were caused by organisms originating in the hospital environment. The most common opportunists were *Pseudomonas aeruginosa, P. spp., Enterobacter cloacae, Hemophilus spp., Candida albicans,* and *Klebsiella spp.* Almost 50 % of adults with leukemia have been found to become carriers of *P. aeruginosa* during the first month of hospitalization [12]. When coupled with the demonstration that the prevalence of gram-negative bacilli among the oropharyngeal flora rises markedly in ill patients during hospital exposure because of impaired pharyngeal clearance mechanisms [13], it becomes readily apparent why these organisms constitute a common cause of oral infections in patients undergoing cancer chemotherapy.

Clinically, there is a high incidence of repeat oral infections with the same organism in the same patient during successive courses of antitumor drug therapy. Even in protected environments like life islands and laminar-air-flow rooms, the oral cavity constitutes a reservoir of microorganisms that can proliferate and produce local and generalized infections. Not only are immunosuppressed patients extremely susceptible to oral infections by common and uncommon pathogens, but they are also prey to saprophytes turned pathogen and to unusual genera and species of microorganisms [14]. Because of their rarity, unusual infection-causing organisms are often dismissed as contaminants, even when isolated directly from mouth lesions. Such neglect may deprive the patient of further anticancer treatment and even of life itself. No organism producing an oral lesion is totally innocuous in this population.

The propensity to oral fungal infections is greatest in patients given antibiotics and steroids in addition to the antitumor agents. Antibiotics have been incriminated as a cause of superinfections with resistant fungi by instigating changes in the oral microbial ecology of the defenseless host. The adrenocortical steroids promote infection with resident oral candida in immunoincompetent subjects by inhibiting inflammation, decreasing capillary permeability, decreasing cellular exudation, interfering with leukocyte migration, causing stabilization of the lysosomal membranes, inhibiting antibody production, and impairing reticuloendothelial function [15].

The more myelosuppressive the chemotherapy protocol, the greater the incidence of oral infections. In a recent study of 1,000 adult patients with acute leukemia or chronic leukemia in the blastic phase treated in hospitals, the oral infection rate was 32.9% [16]. Approximately 50% of the infecting organisms were fungi, 25% gram-negative bacilli, 15% Herpes simplex, and 10% gram-positive cocci. In a companion study [17] of 906 adult inpatients given chemotherapy for solid tumors, the oral infection rate was 9.54%. The distribution of causative organisms in this group was, fungi 66%, gram-negative bacilli 12%, H. simplex 11%, and gram-positive cocci 11%. The difference in frequency of oral infections between the leukemia series and the solid-tumor series is reflective of differences in the degree of myelosuppression and stomatotoxicity. Because leukemia is essentially a myeloproliferative bone-marrow disease, antileukemia chemotherapy protocols are designed to be much more myelosuppressive than those for various types of solid tumors. Antileukemia chemotherapy is also much more stomatotoxic than the antisolid tumor drug combinations and dosages.

The patterns of infection in patients with cancer vary not only with the type of malignancy and degree of loss of host defenses but also with the composition of the chemotherapy [18]. Pus production and abscess formation by pyogenic organisms may be reduced or absent in the presence of profound leucopenia. Corticosteroids used in many anticancer drug combinations may obscure the classic manifestations of microbial infections by lowering fever, reducing the inflammatory response, depressing phagocytosis, altering macrophage migration, and increasing the invasive character of the infectious agents. Unusual patterns or types of oral infections in cancer chemotherapy patients are becoming less and less of a rarity.

CHANGES IN SALIVARY MICROFLORA DURING CANCER CHEMOTHERAPY

Brown, Dreizen, and Bodey studied the changes in the salivary microflora of 12 adult patients with acute leukemia during treatment with POMP (6-mercaptopurine, vincristine, methotrexate, prednisone), COAP (cyclophosphamide, vincristine, cytosine arabinoside, prednisone), or DOAP (daunomycin, vincristine, cytosine arabinoside, prednisone) [19]. Six were given chemotherapy in conventional hospital rooms and six in protected environments. Each had a natural dentition and moderate to good oral hygiene on admission. Those assigned to the protected environments underwent a four-day prior preparation period during which they were given intensive prophylactic treatment with oral and topical antibiotics and with antiseptic agents to eliminate the endogenous microflora. The compositions of the nonabsorbable antibiotic suspensions which were swirled in the mouth for 30 seconds before swallowing, and of the antibiotic ointments applied to the ears, nose, gingiva, groin, and perineum four times daily, are shown in table 4–2. The conventionally hospitalized patients received organism-specific antibiotics only when indicated. Broad-spectrum antibiotics in the form of combinations of either carbenicillin and gentamicin or of carbenicillin and cephalothin were administered whenever the temperature reached 101 °F or above until the causative organisms could be isolated, identified, antibiotic sensitivities determined, and appropriate treatment started.

Table 4–2. Prophylactic antibiotic regimens for protected environments

Oral regimens

Antibiotics	Dosage
Antibacterial agents	
Regimen A	
Paromomycin sulfate	500 mg
Polymyxin B sulfate	70 mg
Vancomycin hydrochloride	250 mg
Regimen B	
Gentamicin sulfate[1]	200 mg
Vancomycin hydrochloride	250 mg
Antifungal agents	
Amphotericin B[2]	500 mg
Nystatin	3.6 million units

All antibiotics except nystatin were given in flavored solution every 4 hours. Nystatin was given as 6 tablets and 6 cc suspension every 4 hours.

Topical regimens

Antibiotics	Spray (cc)	Concentration in ointment (g)	Gel (g)
Neomycin sulfate	100 mg	50 mg	100 mg
Nystatin	—	25,000 units	50,000 units
Vancomycin hydrochloride	10 mg	5 mg	10 mg
Polymyxin B sulfate	5 mg	2.5 mg	5 mg

[1]Supplied by Schering Corp. as Garamycin syrup.
[2]Supplied by E. R. Squibb and Sons as Preparation AJS.

Residual whole saliva was obtained from the floor of the mouth by means of a sterile wire loop and stimulated whole saliva by the chewing of sterile rubber bands. Specimens were collected in the morning before breakfast, daily mouth care, and oral medications. All patients were sampled at least twice before treatment was started and at least once a week throughout the hospital stay. Aliquots of each sample were examined microscopically and the remainder processed and plated on selective media for isolation and enumeration of the microbial categories listed in table 4–3. Species and strain differentiations were made for isolates considered unique or reflective of a significant change in the oral flora.

Microscopic examination of the samples of whole saliva obtained during chemotherapy for leukemia in protected and conventional hospital environments disclosed the presence of massive numbers of desquamated epithelial cells. Many of the smears contained blastospores and pseudohyphae of *Candida* (figure 4–1). Oral spirochetes were rarely found during antileukemia treatment and were never seen after antibiotic therapy. Protozoa (amoeba or *Trichomonas*) were not detected in the salivas of any of the patients studied.

There were distinctive quantitative changes in the counts of cultivable salivary organisms in the conventionally hospitalized patients given the immunosuppressive and myelosuppressive antileukemia drugs. The qualitative and quantitative differences are graphed in figure

Table 4–3. Selective Media for Isolation of Saliva and Plaque Microflora

Stimulated and residual whole saliva		Coronal dental plaque 2.4 ± 0.4 mg
	Microbial enumeration and identification	
Aerobic cultures: 2–3 days at 37°C		Anaerobic cultures: Displacement (95% N_2–5% CO_2)[1], Gaspak & Brewer (95% H_2–5% CO_2): 3–7 days at 37°C
	Plating media and microbial categories enumerated	
Total Aerobes Neisseria	Heart infusion agar with defibrinated horse blood (5%)	Total anaerobes, diphtheroids (catalase +. −)
Streptococcus salivarius *S. sanguis* *S. mitis*	Mitis salivarius agar plus tellurite and with or without bacitracin and 20% sucrose	*S. mutans* 18–24 hr. anaerobically; 24 hr. room temperature
Staphylococci	Staphylococcus 110 agar	
	Veillonella agar with Tween 80 and vancomycin	Veillonella
Lactobacilli Hemofermentative Heterofermentative	Rogosa SL agar with glacial acetic acid	
	Trypticase soy agar[2] with crystal violet and vancomycin	Fusobacteria
Yeast	Sabouraud—Dextrose agar	
	Heart infusion agar with laked blood, menadione, $NaHCO_3$, kanamycin, and vancomycin	Bacteroides
Enterics	Desoxycholate agar	
	PPLO Agar and heart infusion agar yeast extract sol., horse serum, thallium acetate, and penicillin	Mycoplasma

[1]Steel wool coated with acidified copper sulfate solution.
[2]BBL; other media-Difco.

4–2. All microbial counts increased appreciably following five-day courses of chemotherapy except for fusobacteria, which underwent a notable decline. All counts possibly affected by antibiotic medication to combat infection were excluded from the computations. Median rather than mean counts were used to eliminate the impact of extremely low or high numbers. The increases were suggestive of drug-induced immunosuppression. The decrease in fusobacteria may have been caused by one or more of the antileukemia drugs since these organisms are very sensitive to agents like methotrexate.

The effects of prophylactic and therapeutic antibiotics on the salivary microflora of the 12 patients receiving antileukemia chemotherapy are summarized in figure 4–3. Topical application of the antibiotic prophylactic regimens for the patients in the protected environments greatly reduced all of the microorganisms monitored except *Lactobacilli.* Systemically administered therapeutic antibiotics such as gentamicin, cephalothin, and/or carbenicillin, for suspected or proven infections, produced marked reductions in *Streptococci, Fusobacteria,* and *Neisseria.* These antibiotics failed to lower the saliva levels of *Lactobaccilli* and *Bacteroides* and only reduced the concentration of total anaerobes, total aerobes, and *Veillonella* by 25% or less.

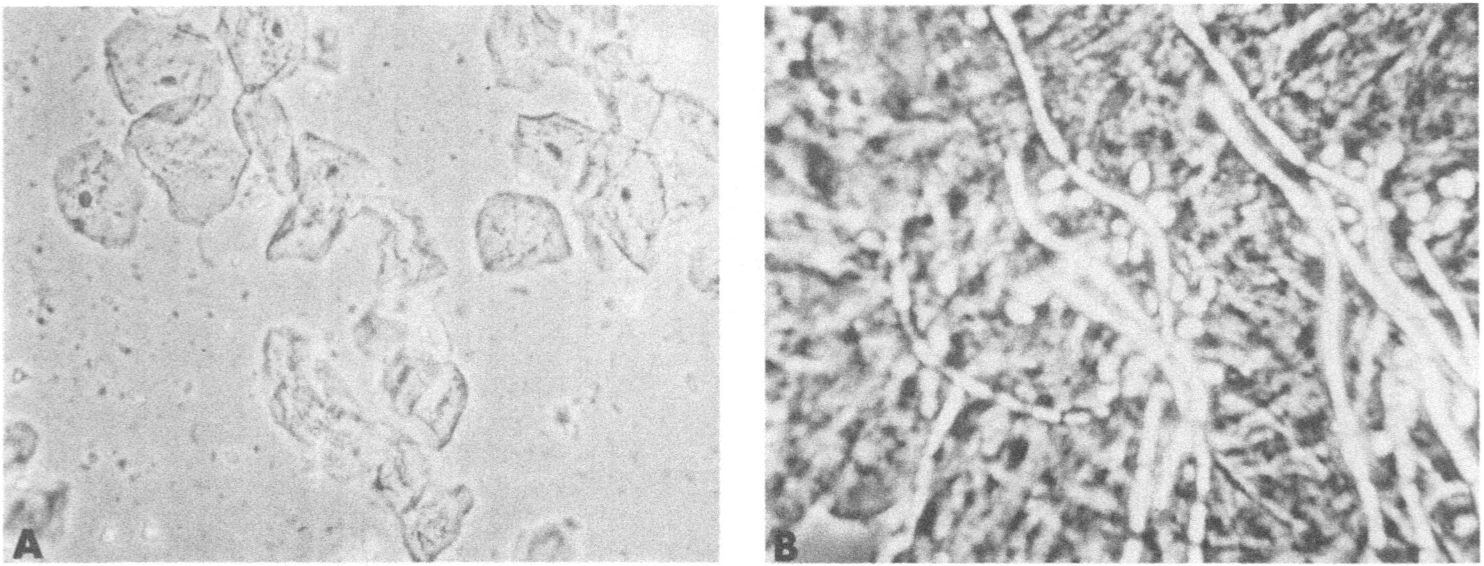

Figure 4–1. Microscopic appearance of stimulated whole saliva collected from a patient undergoing antileukemia chemotherapy. **A:** masses of epithelial cells following drug-induced desquamation (×100). **B:** clumps of blastospores and pseudohyphae of *C. spp.* (×400).

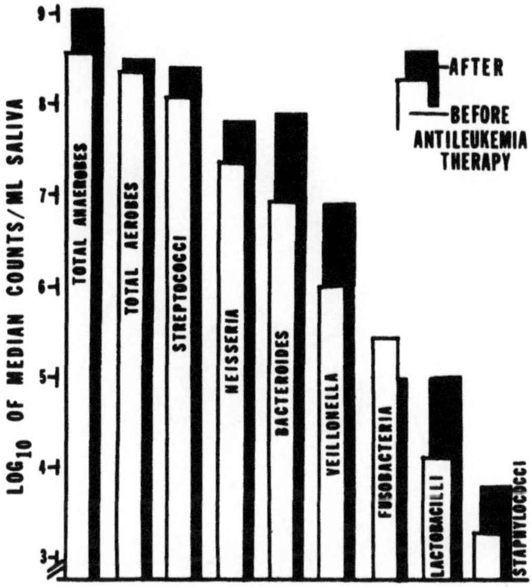

Figure 4–2. Comparison of median counts of cultivable microorganisms from stimulated whole saliva before and after five-day courses of antileukemic chemotherapy.

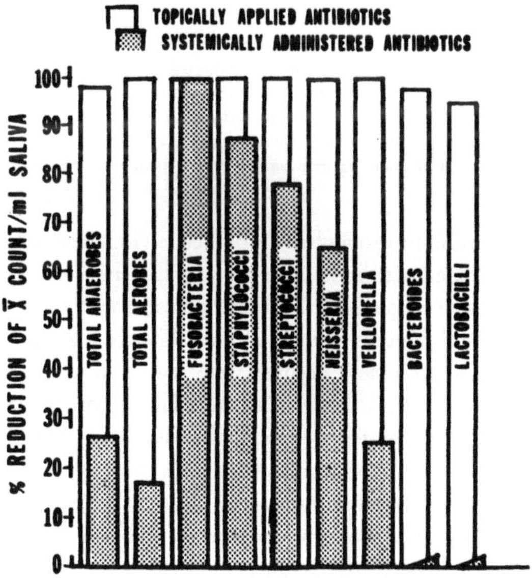

Figure 4–3. Comparative effects of prophylactic oral doses of nonabsorbable and systemically administered broad-spectrum antibiotics on cultivable microorganisms in stimulated whole saliva.

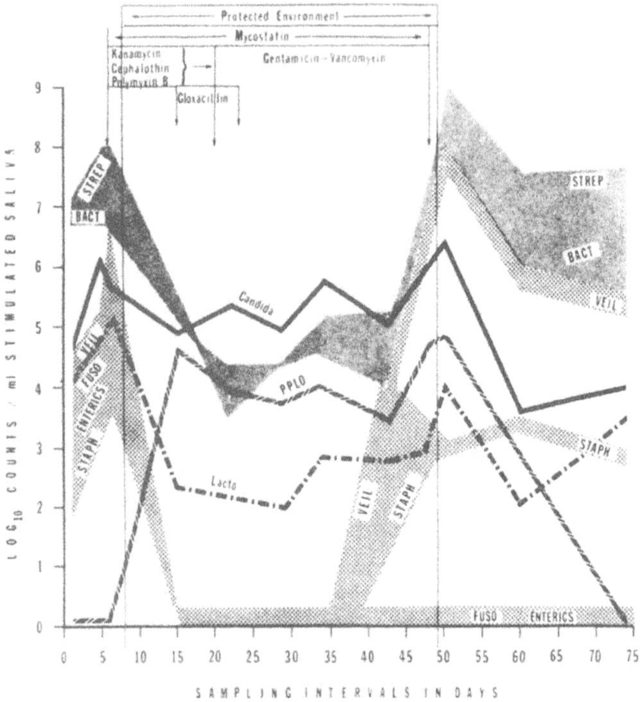

Figure 4–4. Changes in saliva microbial profile of a protected environment patient with acute myelogenous leukemia receiving chemotherapy, antibiotic prophylactic regimens, and systemic antibiotic treatment to combat infections. STREP = total streptococci; VEIL = *Veillonella;* LACTO = lactobacilli; BACT = bacteroides; PPLO = *Mycoplasma;* FUSO = fusobacteria; STAPH = salt-tolerant staphylococci; ENTERICS = mixed genera of gram-negative aerobic bacilli commonly recoverable from feces.

The influence of antibiotic prophylaxis, protected environment, and immunosuppressive drug therapy in a patient with acute myelogenous leukemia is illustrated in figure 4–4. Combining the intensive prophylactic antibiotic protocol with the protected environment resulted in a pronounced diminution in all of the cultivable organisms except *Candida* and *Mycoplasma.* The most prominent declines were registered by *S. salivarius, Veillonella, Fusobacteria,* and *Staphylococci.* Although both procedures generally suppressed the total oral microflora, neither completely sterilized the oral cavity. Many organisms like *Streptococci, Bacteroides,* and *Lactobacilli* not only survived attempts at complete eradication but persisted in the mouth at relatively high levels throughout the study period. In contrast, only *Candida* and *Klebsiella* were recovered from the oropharynx and only *Escherichia coli* was found in the stool of this patient during treatment in a laminar-air-flow room. The effect of immunosuppressive chemotherapy and consequent loss of the immune restraints on the oral microflora was vividly demonstrated by the sharp rise in salivary *Streptococci, Bacteroides, Lactobacilli,* and *Candida* that followed termination of the antibiotics while the patient was still in the protected environment. These counts reverted to pretreatment levels after

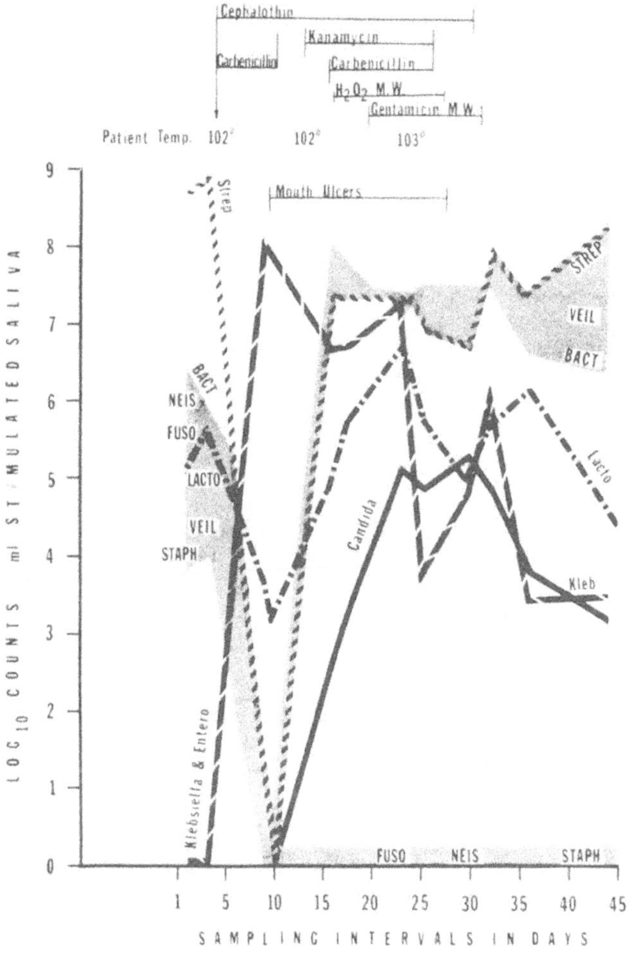

Figure 4–5. Changes in saliva microbial profile of a conventionally hospitalized patient with acute myelogenous leukemia receiving cancer chemotherapy and antibiotics for a *K. pneumoniae* oral superinfection. STREP = total streptococci; BACT = bacteroides; NEIS = *Neisseria;* FUSO = fusobacteria; LACTO = lactobacilli; VEIL = *Veillonella;* STAPH = salt-tolerant staphylococci; KLEB = *Klebsiella;* ENTERO = *Enterobacter.* Mouthwashes listed as M.W.

completion of chemotherapy and release of the patient from the laminar-air-flow room.

Four of the six patients treated for acute myelogenous leukemia in regular hospital rooms showed a precipitous increase in one of the oral organisms that led to an extensive mouth infection in one and reflected fulminating septicemias in three. The oral microbial profile of the patient who developed an oral superinfection by *K. pneumoniae* involving the gingival, palatal, lingual, and labial mucosa subsequent to receiving antibiotics for a fever of unknown origin is shown in figure 4–5. All of the oral microflora except for *Lactobacilli*

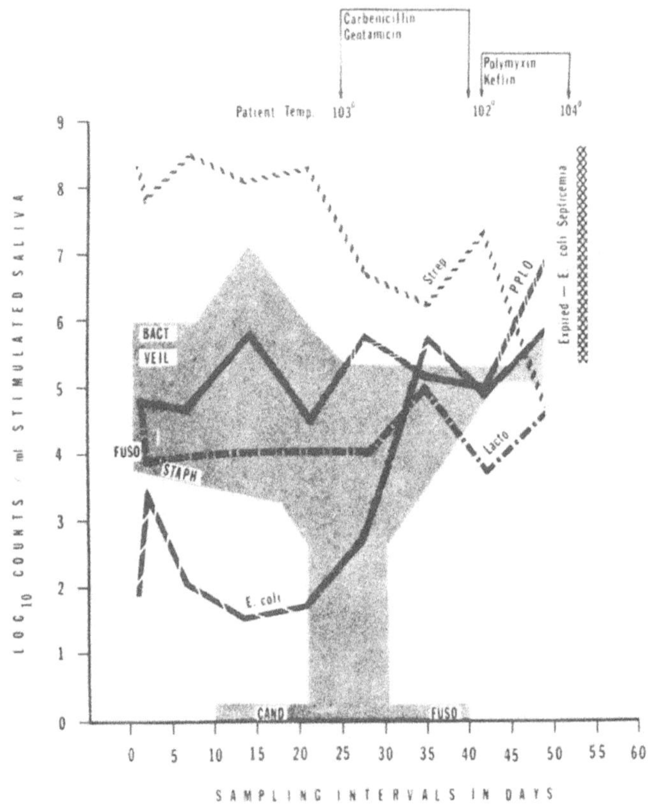

Figure 4–6. Changes in saliva microbial profile of a conventionally hospitalized patient with acute myelogenous leukemia who died from *E. coli* septicemia during chemotherapy. STREP = total streptococci; BACT = bacteroides; VEIL = *Veillonella;* FUSO = fusobacteria; STAPH = salt-tolerant staphylococci; CAND = *Candida spp.;* LACTO = lactobacilli; PPLO = *Mycoplasma.*

were replaced by *Enterobacter-Klebsiella* organisms for more than three days. The administration of specific antibiotics against *K. pneumoniae* was accompanied by an increase in *C. albicans* from an undetectable level to approximately 10,000 colony-forming units per milliliter of saliva. Changes in the oral microflora of the patients who developed *E. coli, P. aeruginosa,* and *C. albicans* septicemias are graphed in figures 4–6, 4–7, and 4–8. Increasing numbers of *E. coli, P. aeruginosa,* and *C. albicans* were recovered from the respective salivas beginning three weeks antemortem for *E. coli,* four weeks antemortem for *P. aeruginosa,* and other enterics and two weeks antemortem for *C. albicans.*

Persons with acute leukemia have essentially normal antibody responses, delayed hypersensitivity reactions, and serum immunoglobulin levels. Although the leukemic process does not alter the phagocytic action of mature granulocytes, the disease prompts formation of large numbers of blast cells and immature granulocytes with little or no phagocytic or digestive action. The noteworthy increments in many members of the oral microbial

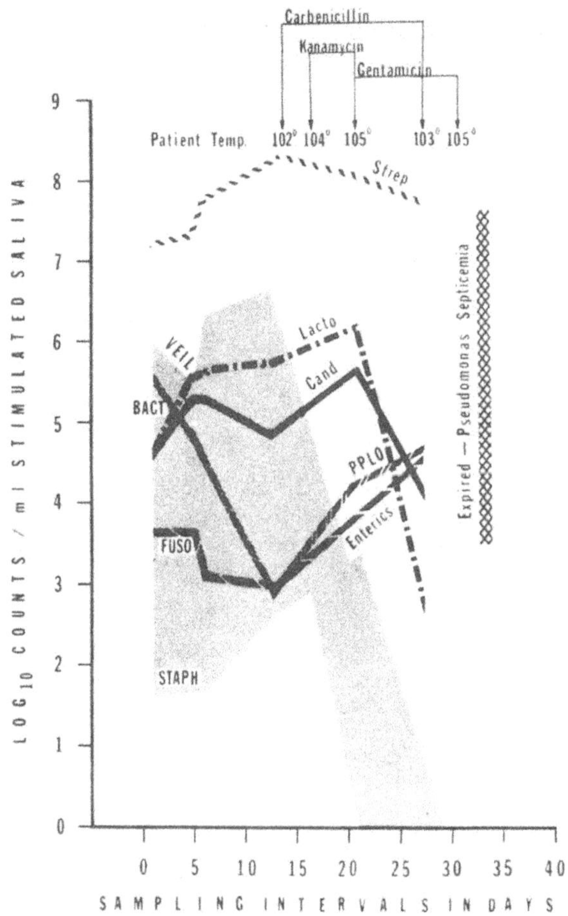

Figure 4–7. Changes in saliva microbial profile of a conventionally hospitalized patient with acute myelogenous leukemia who died from *P. aeruginosa* septicemia. STREP = total streptococci; VEIL = *Veillonella;* LACTO = lactobacilli; BACT = bacteroides; PPLO = *Mycoplasma;* FUSO = fusobacteria; STAPH = salt-tolerant staphylococci; ENTERICS = mixed genera of gram-negative aerobic bacilli commonly recoverable from feces.

population that occurs during chemotherapy for acute leukemia, the intraoral establishment of exogenous bacteria that replace endogenous flora, and the initiation of oral infections by some normally saprophytic organisms all point to suppression of cellular and humoral immune mechanisms in these patients by the antitumor drugs. Such drug-induced immunosuppression chain-linked with drug and disease precipitated myelosuppression and drug-provoked oral mucositis makes the mouth of the patient on cancer chemotherapy an unusually fertile field for infection whether treated in a conventional or protected environment.

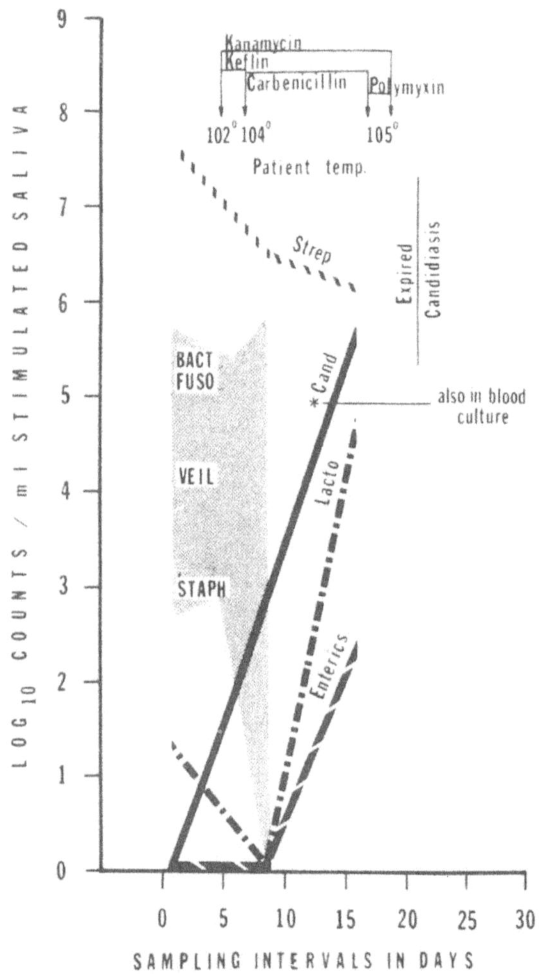

Figure 4–8. Changes in saliva microbial profile of a conventionally hospitalized patient with acute myelogenous leukemia who died from a *C. albicans* septicemia during chemotherapy. STREP = total streptococci; BACT = bacteroides; FUSO = fusobacteria; VEIL = *Veillonella;* STAPH = salt-tolerant staphylococci; LACT = lactobacilli; CAND = *Candida spp.;* ENTERICS = mixed genera of gram-negative aerobic bacilli commonly recoverable from feces.

CHANGES IN PLAQUE MICROFLORA DURING CANCER CHEMOTHERAPY

Subsequent studies by Brown and associates [20] and by Wheatcroft and others [21] focused on the effects of immunosuppressive chemotherapy and of antibiotics on the microbial composition of dental plaque in cancer patients. The culturable plaque microflora of six patients with acute leukemia and of six patients with residual or metastatic solid tumors (3, breast cancer; 1, lymphocytic lymphoma; 1, leiomyosarcoma; 1, adenocarcinoma of lung) was monitored during remission-induction and maintenance chemotherapy. Six patients (3, leukemia; 3, solid tumor) were treated in laminar-air-flow-protected environments and six (3, leukemia; 3, solid tumor) in nonprotected hospital environments. Protected-environment patients received an intensive prophylactic antibiotic regimen whereas the conventional environment patients were given antibiotics only when indicated. Patient-centered chemotherapy was administered intermittently in combinations of three to five drugs depending on the type of malignancy. The specific chemotherapy drug protocols and the prophylactic and therapeutic antibiotics to which the subjects were exposed are detailed in table 4–4.

Pooled coronal plaque samples of 2.4 ± 0.4 mg were collected at least twice before institution of chemotherapy and at weekly intervals thereafter throughout the hospitalization period. A small aliquot was used for phase contrast cinemicrographic examination and the remainder was processed for plating on selective media for cultivation and enumeration of 21 microbial categories (table 4–3). Phase contrast cinemicrography enabled observation of both culturable and nonculturable plaque organisms. Slides were prepared from undiluted plaque and photographed with a Bolex camera through a Reichert anoptral phase microscope.

Plaque levels of most of the plateable organisms were comparable in the conventional and protected environment patients with either solid tumors or acute leukemia prior to chemotherapy. As shown in figure 4–9, most plaque microbial counts were higher in the patients receiving antileukemia therapy than in those treated for solid tumors. Except for *Candida,* plaque microbial concentrations in the solid tumor patients tended to decrease during the anticancer treatment while those in the patients with leukemia remained fairly constant during the same period. Plaque numbers of *C. spp.* increased in both groups of patients, attaining the highest values in the solid-tumor patients with the lowest bacterial counts.

The plaque microbial changes in protected environment patients receiving chemotherapy for solid tumors and for acute leukemia are compared in figure 4–10. Plaque counts of all designated microbial categories except *Candida* declined sharply in response to antibiotic prophylaxis and protected-environment isolation. The changes were significantly greater in the leukemia than in the solid-tumor group. The diminished numbers persisted until termination of the cancer treatment, after which they gradually returned to near-pretreatment values.

A comparison of the influence of the antitumor treatment environment on the cultivable plaque microorganisms of the solid-tumor and leukemia patients is shown in figures 4–11 and 4–12. Plaque counts of *C. spp.* increased in both the protected and conventional environments. The increments in the protected-environment patients significantly exceeded those in the conventionally hospitalized group. Rise in *Candida* was accompanied by significant decrements in all plaque bacterial counts in the protected environment patients and by imperceptible to minor decreases in the nonprotected patients.

The impact of oral and systemic antibiotics on the plaque microbial population is shown in figure 4–13. Topically applied antibiotics greatly reduced the counts of the plaque organisms with the notable exceptions of *Bacteroides, Mycoplasma, Lactobacilli,* and enteric *Bacilli.* These shifts were paralleled by marked increases in plaque *Candida.* Systemically

Table 4–4. Cancer chemotherapy and antibiotic treatment of patients in protected and conventional environments

Sex	Age	Diagnosis	Chemotherapy	Antibiotic prophylaxis	Systemic antibiotic
			Protected Environment		
F	37	AML	Ad-OAP	Standard PE regimen	Bactrim
F	44	AMML	Adriamycin	Tobramycin–vancomycin solution	Carbenicillin
M	39	AMML	Vincristine	Nilstat–nystatin	Cefamandole
			Cytosine arabinoside	5–fluorocytosine	Cloxacillin
			Prednisone	Germicidal soap bath and shampoo	Colistin
				NNVP ointment[1]	Keflin
				NNVP rectal gel	Mezlocillin
				NVP nasal spray[2]	Netilmicin
				NVP throat spray	Ticarcillin
		Adenocarcinoma	FAC	Leukemia patients	
F	52	Breast	5–fluorouracil	Cefazolin–colistimethate	
F	55	Breast	Adriamycin	Chloramphenicol–amphotericin B	
F	34	Breast	Cyclophosphamide	Ampicillin–tobramycin	
				Clindamycin–amphotericin B	

Table 4–4 (continued)

			Conventional Environment	
F	24	ALL	CHOP-Bleo	Ampicillin
F	39	ALL	Cyclophosphamide	Bactrim
M	33	ALL	Adriamycin	Carbenicillin
			Vincristine	Cephradine
			Prednisone	Keflin
			Bleomycin	Mezlocillin
F	51	Lymphoma Abdomen	CTX-BCNU-VP_{16}	Miconazole
			CTX (cyclophosphamide)	Netilmicin
			BCNU (carmustine)	Penicillin G
			VP_{16} (etoposide)	Ticarcillin
				Tobramycin
M	63	Leiomyosarcoma Colon	Cyvadic	
			Cyclophosphamide	
			Vincristine	
			Adriamycin	
			Dacarbazine	
F	45	Adenocarcinoma Lung	FACP-AMSA	
			Ftorufur Cyclophosphamide	
			Adriamycin Cis Platinum	
			AMSA (adridinyl anisidide)	

[1]Neomycin-nystatin-vancomycin-polymyxin B.
[2]Nystatin-vancomycin-polymixin B.

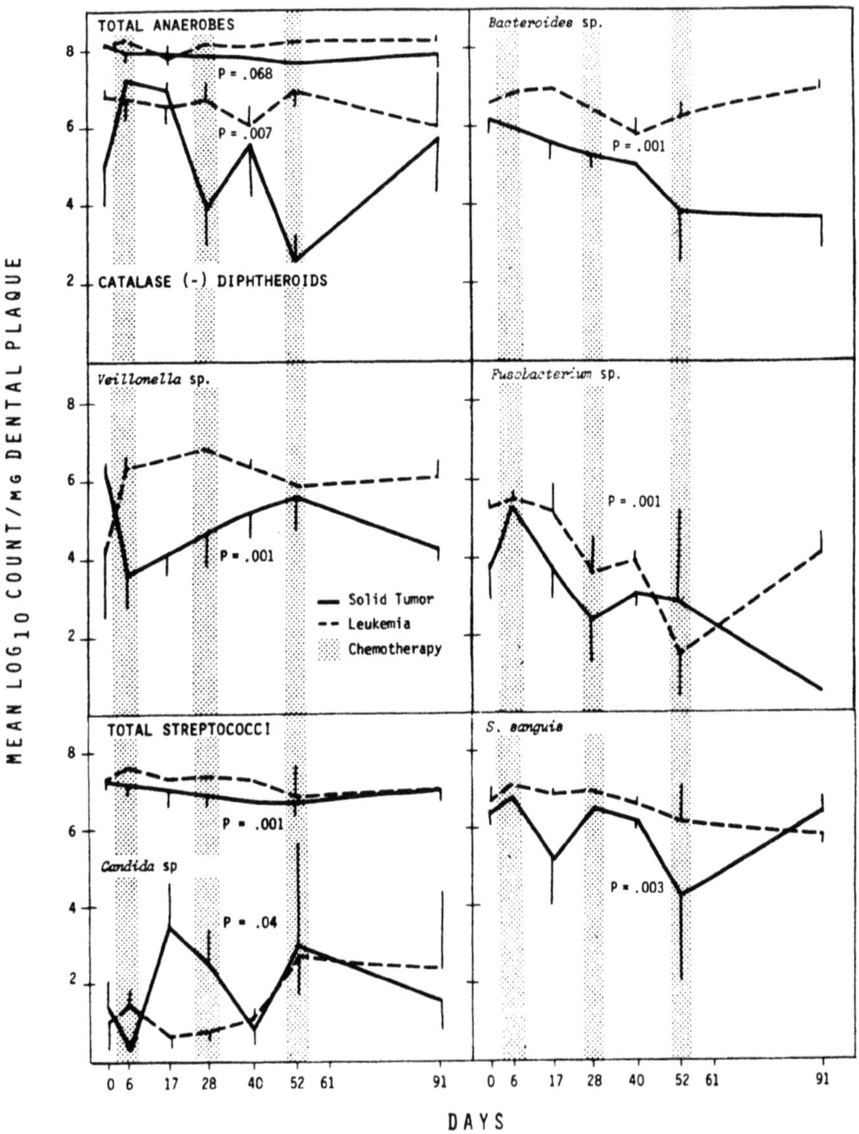

Figure 4–9. Plaque microbial changes in conventional environment patients receiving chemotherapy for solid tumors compared to those treated for leukemia under similar conditions.

administered antibiotics given along with the topical agents had an additive effect on some organisms further depressing total anaerobes, total diphtheroids, catalase-negative diphtheroids, *Bacteroides,* and *Veillonella.*

The individual plaque microbial profiles of a patient with acute leukemia treated in a laminar-air-flow room and of a similar patient treated in a conventional-hospital environ-

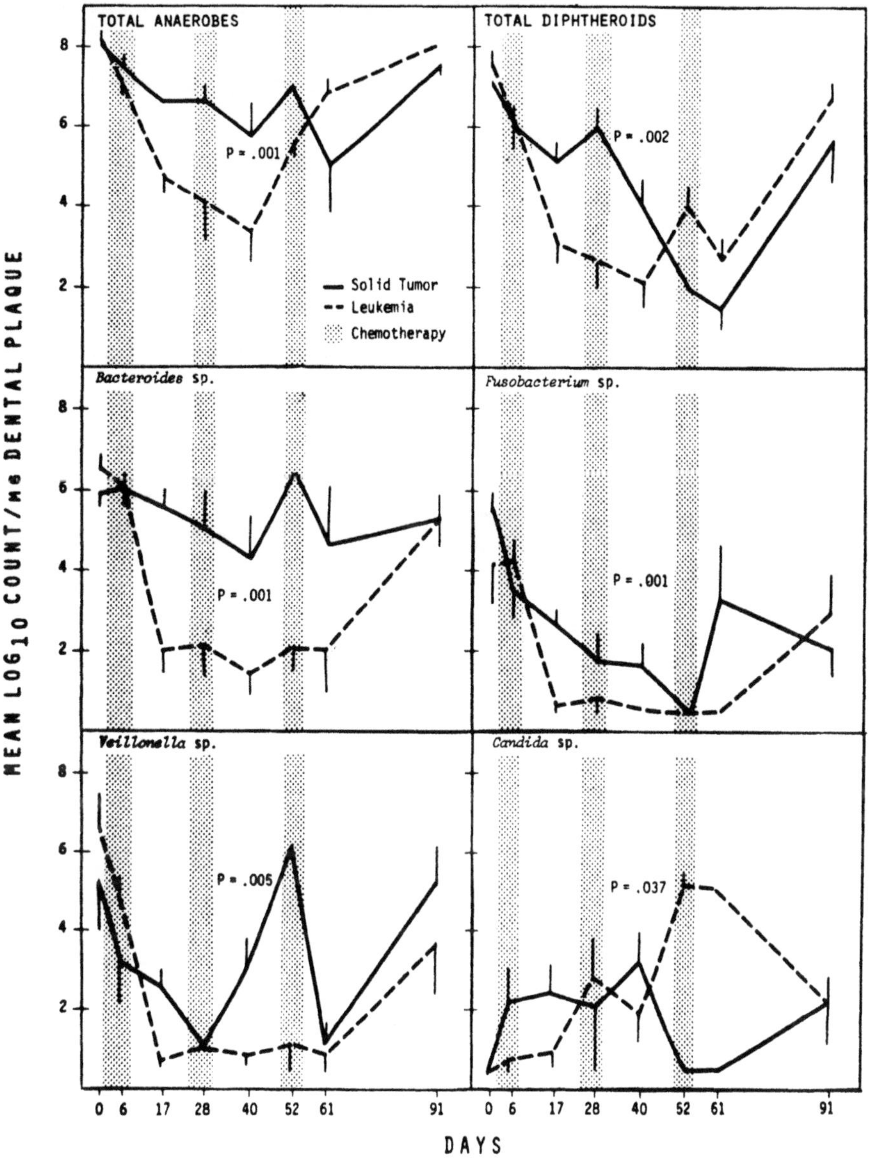

Figure 4–10. Plaque microbial changes in protected environment patients receiving chemotherapy for solid tumors and for leukemia.

ment are shown in figure 4–14. Total *Streptococci,* total diphtheroids, and several other organisms decreased by 4 to 6 log_{10} units while *C. spp* rose appreciably in the protected-environment patient. These changes were largely attributable to the prophylactic antibiotic protocol since most of the counts returned to pretreatment levels when the antibiotics were

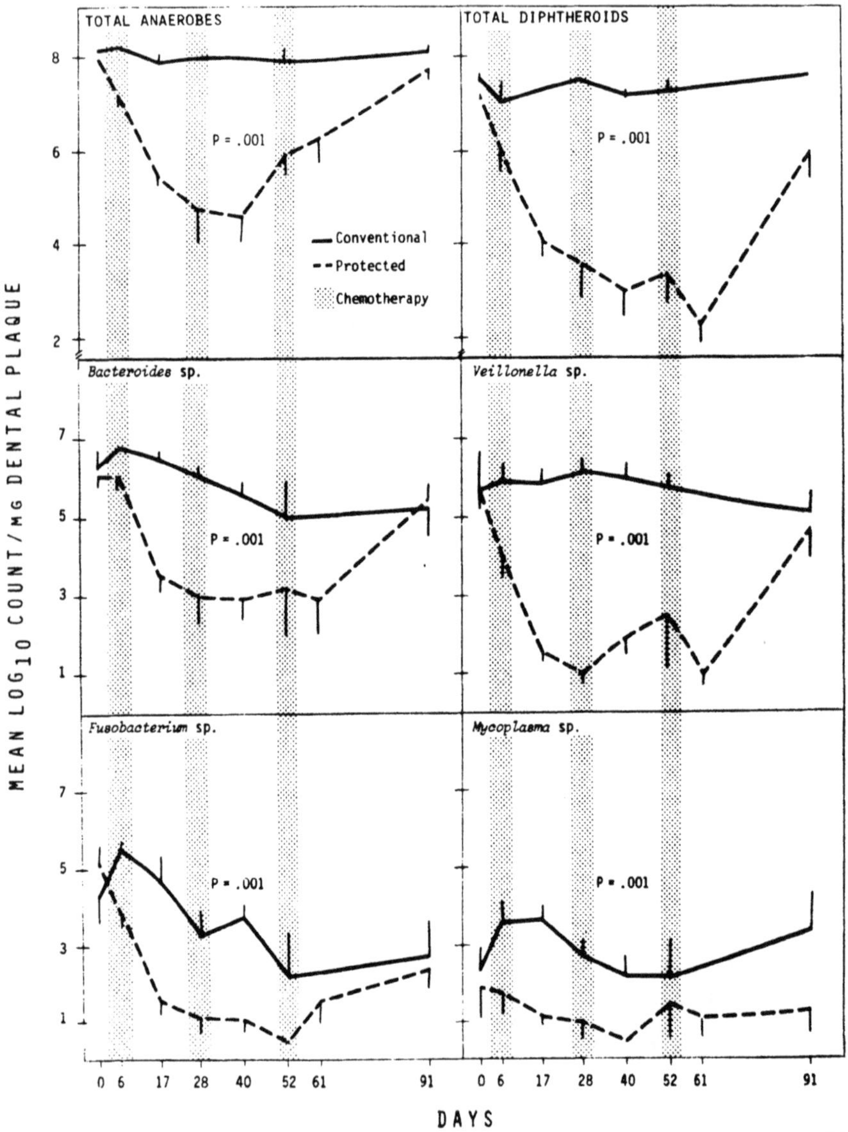

Figure 4–11. Changes in plaque anaerobes in patients treated in protected environment compared to those treated in conventional environment.

discontinued. In contrast, most of the plaque counts stayed relatively constant in the patient treated out of the protected environment. Changes were limited to decreases in plaque *S. mutans, S. salivarius, Lactobacilli,* and *Fusobacteria* and to a rise in *C. spp.* whenever systemic antibiotics were given to combat intervening infections.

The cinemicrographic profiles of the plaque microflora showed dramatic decreases in all

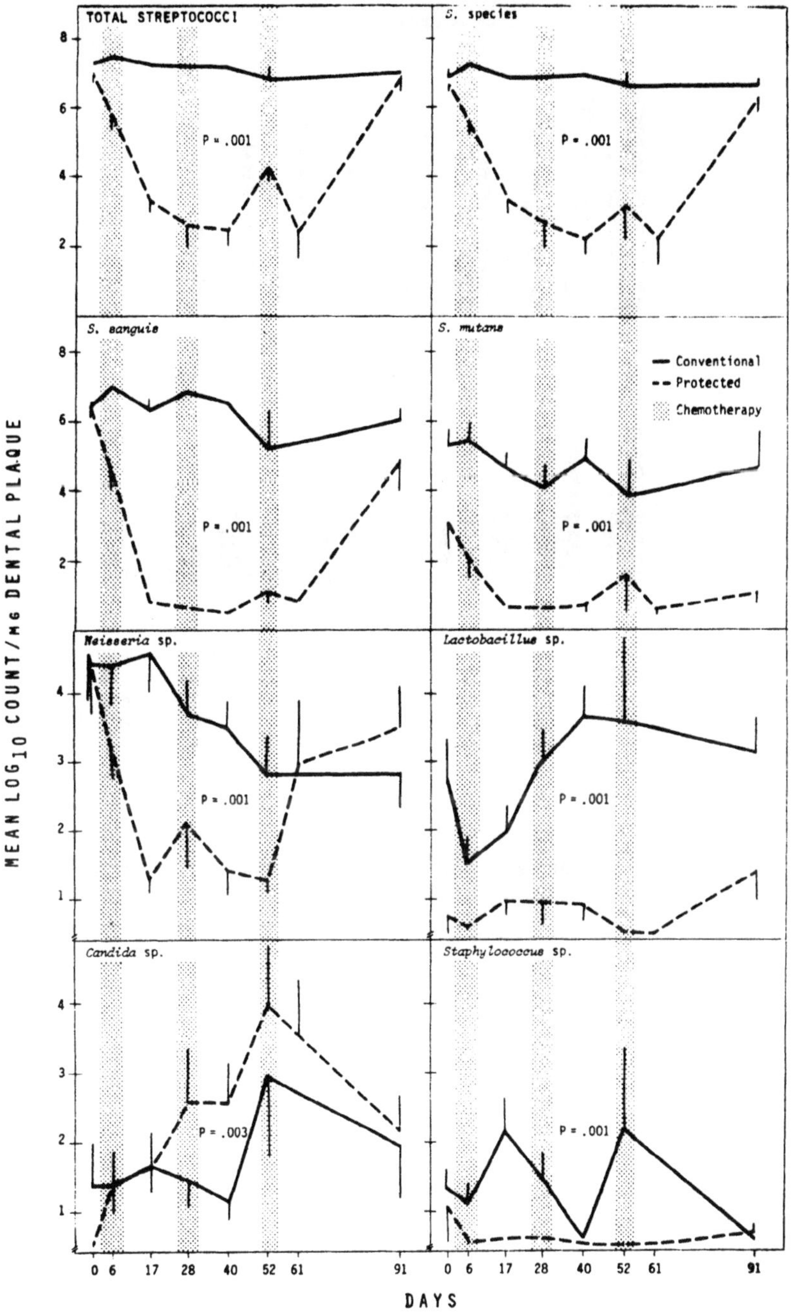

Figure 4–12. Changes in plaque streptococci, *Neisseria,* lactobacilli, staphylococci, and *Candida* in patients treated in protected and conventional environments.

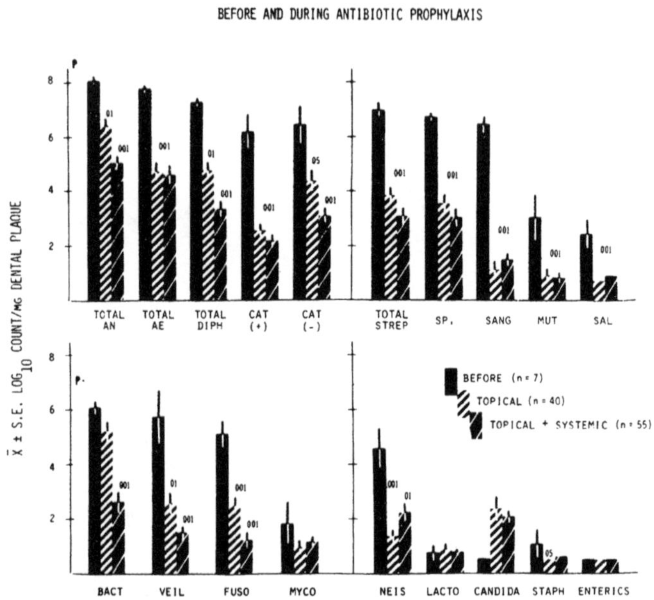

Figure 4–13. Comparison of plaque microbial levels before and after administration of prophylactic oral and of oral plus systemic antibiotics. An = anaerobes; Ae = aerobes; Diph = diphtheroids; CAT (+) = catalase positive diphtheroids; CAT (−) = catalase negative diphtheroids; Strep = streptococci; sp = unidentified streptococci; Sang = *S. sanguis;* Mut = *S. mutans;* Sal = *S. salivarius;* Bact = bacteroides; Veil = *Veillonella;* Fuso = fusobacteria; Myco = *Mycoplasma;* Neis = *Neisseria;* Lacto = lactobacilli; *Candida* = *Candida;* Staph = staphylococci; Enterics = gram-negative aerobic enteric bacilli.

morphologic types in the patients treated in the protected environments. Neither the laminar-air-flow rooms nor the multiple prophylactic antibiotics, however, completely eliminated all of the plaque organisms. In the patients so treated the plaques were converted from complex microbial microcosms to sparse collections of rods, cocci, and/or filaments.

CLINICAL CHARACTERISTICS OF CHEMOTHERAPY-ASSOCIATED ORAL INFECTIONS

Surveys of infections in patients receiving cancer chemotherapy have identified the mouth, respiratory tract, urinary tract, hepatobiliary tract, anorectal area, and skin as the organ sites most frequently involved [11,22,23]. Mouth infections in these patients range from surface colonization of the mucosa through superficial and deep ulceration, cellulitis and necrosis, to perforation of the underlying structures. Approximately one in five represent polyinfections by two or more microorganisms, most often *Candida* and herpes [16]. The most common infection sites are the lips and tongue followed frequently by the buccal mucosa, gingiva, palate, and oropharynx and occasionally by the major salivary glands. Both the keratinized and nonkeratinized components of the mucosa appear to be equally susceptible. The lesions range in color from white through yellow, red and purple, to black; in number, from single to multitudinous and in character from discrete to diffuse. Symptomatically,

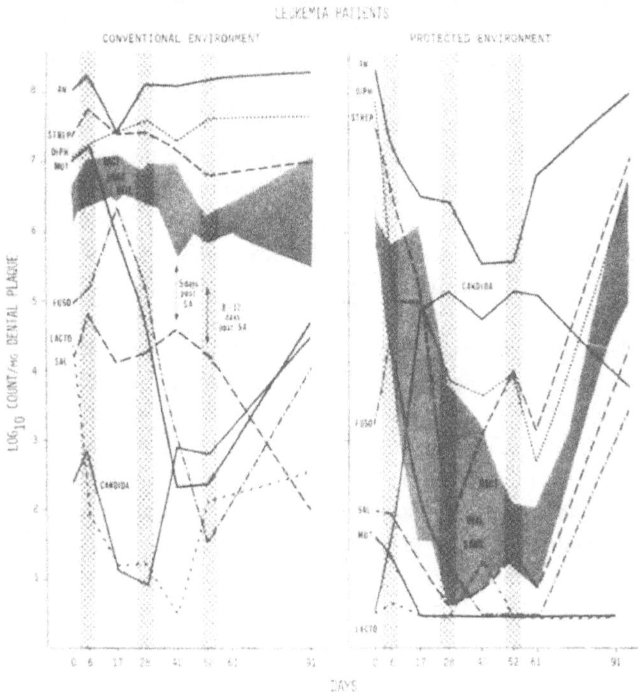

Figure 4–14. Plaque microbial profile of a patient with leukemia treated in a conventional environment and of a patient with leukemia treated in a protected environment.

they are productive of discomfort, burning, pain, dysphagia, fever, anorexia, and malaise —the degree dependent on the nature of the infection and on the extent of involvement. None of the lesions are pathognomonic per se. Documentation of the etiologic agent requires recovery, isolation, and speciation of the organism or organisms by appropriate cultural, biochemical, and microscopic procedures.

Fungal infections

Candidiasis

As previously mentioned, *C. spp.* are responsible for approximately one-half of all oral infections that arise during antileukemia chemotherapy and for almost two-thirds of those that occur in patients given antineoplastic drugs for solid tumors. *Candida* is part of the normal human oral microflora in at least 50% of the population. Of the more than 80 species in this genus only seven, *(C. albicans, C. tropicalis, C. parapsilosis, C. guilliermondii, C. pseudotropicalis, C. krusei,* and *C. stellatoidea)* are regularly cultured from man with *C. albicans* by far the most common. These usually harmless human commensals become pathogenic when the host defense mechanisms are disrupted by the cytotoxic, immunosuppressive, and myelosuppressive anticancer drugs. Host defenses that appear to be most important against the development of candidiasis are adequate numbers of circulating neutrophils and a normal lymphocyte-monocyte interaction, both of which are depressed by antineoplastic drugs. Antibiotic treatment for bacterial infections also greatly increase the risk of candida infections in such patients.

The most frequent sites of oral candidiasis are the dorsum, sides, and undersurface of the tongue, buccal, gingival, palatal, and pharyngeal mucosa and the commissures of the lips. Candidal colonization is manifested by elevated, creamy-white, curd-like strands, beads, flecks, and/or patches that adhere to the underlying mucosa. The longer the duration of the infection, the greater the tendency for colony coalescence that may blanket large expanses of the mucosa. The fungal growth contributes to the formation of a pseudomembrane comprised of masses of hyphae, pseudohyphae, and yeast forms, desquamated epithelial cells, leukocytes, bacteria, necrotic tissue, and food debris. Removal of the pseudomembrane by scraping exposes a painful, raw, superficially ulcerated, bleeding mucosal surface. The white patches are often discolored by tobacco smoke and/or food stains. Examples of a gingival infection by *C. albicans* that developed in a patient with adenocarcinoma of the breast in a protected environment and of paradontal, lingual, and palatal infections by the same organism in hospitalized adults receiving antileukemia chemotherapy are shown in figure 4–15. The great dangers of oral candidiasis in such patients are esophageal infection from swallowing the organisms that produces severe dysphagia and substernal chest pain and oral or esophageal mucosal penetration that leads to septicemia and widespread hematogenous dissemination.

The drugs of choice for controlling oral infections are listed in table 4–5. Mild oral candidiasis can be treated with topical preparations of nystatin or clotrimazole. Nystatin is most effective when administered by mouth as a vaginal tablet containing 100,000 units of drug six times a day. The tablet is allowed to melt in the mouth slowly and the contents swallowed. Clotrimazole is given as a dissolvable oral troche containing 10 mg of drug three to six times a day. Severe infections not responsive to the topical agents must be treated with a daily dose of 20 to 30 mg amphotericin B infused intravenously. Care must be taken to monitor renal function as amphotericin B is potentially nephrotoxic.

Aspergillosis:

Aspergillosis is second only to candidiasis in frequency of mycoses among immunocompromised cancer patients. Hospital air has been found to contain *Aspergillus fumigatus, A. flavus, A. niger,* and other species. The organisms are usually acquired by inhalation of airborne spores that germinate in a mucus medium. The vegetative forms have a propensity to invade the mucosa, underlying connective tissue, and bone. They penetrate into the walls of the regional blood vessels where they proliferate and trigger thrombosis, infarction, and necrosis.

Oral aspergillosis in patients on cancer chemotherapy often involves the palate where the lesions present as extremely painful, yellowish erosive ulcers surrounded by a black border. As shown in figure 4–16**A**, the mouth can be involved by direct extension of infections originating in the paranasal sinuses. In this patient with acute myelogenous leukemia, *A. fumigatus* caused a fulminating noma-like gangrenous necrosis that consumed a large part of the ala nasi, philtrum, lips, and left cheek. Oral aspergillosis is best treated

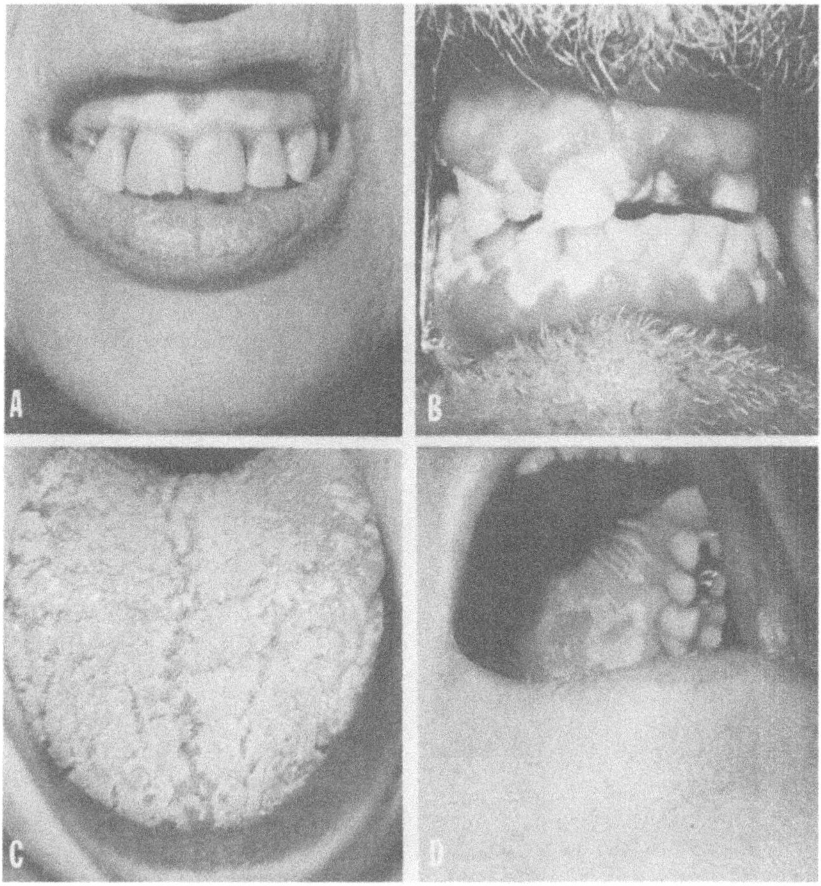

Figure 4–15. Oral *C. albicans* infections in patients undergoing cancer chemotherapy.

A. Candidal infection of gingiva in patient treated in protected environment for adenocarcinoma of breast.
B. Paradontal candidiasis in patient with acute myelomonocytic leukemia.
C. Lingual candidiasis in patient with acute myelogenous leukemia.
D. Palatal candidiasis in patient with adenocarcinoma of breast.

with amphotericin B. Such treatment is only successful, however, in patients who have achieved complete remission of the malignancy.

Mucormycosis

Mucormycosis is a much less frequently encountered infectious complication of cytoreductive chemotherapy than is either candidiasis or aspergillosis. The most common etiologic agents are members of the genera *Rhizopus, Absidia,* and *Mucor.* Oral involvement occurs almost exclusively in the form of rhinocerebral mucormycosis. The infection begins in

Table 4–5. Antimicrobial drugs of choice for cancer chemotherapy-associated oral infections

Infection	Drug	Usual dose
Staphylococcus aureus	Methicillin	1 g q.6h. iv
S. epidermidis	Penicillin G	600,000 units q.4h. iv
	Vancomycin	500 mg q.6h. iv
	Rifampin	600 mg q.d. po
Streptococcus faecalis	Penicillin G	
	Gentamicin	50 mg/M² q.6h. iv
S. pyogenes	Penicillin G	
Herpes simplex	0.5% Idoxuridine	Topical
	3% Vidarabine	Topical
Candida	Nystatin	100,000 units (vaginal tab) × 6 q.d. po
	Clotrimazole	10 mg (oral troche) × 3–6 q.d. po
	Amphotericin B	20–30 mg q.d. iv
Pseudomonas	Ticarcillin	4 g q.4h. iv
	Carbenicillin	5 g q.4h. iv
	Aminoglycoside	
	Tobramycin	50 mg/M² q.6h. iv
	Gentamicin	50 mg/M² q.6h. iv
	Amikacin	150 mg/M² q.6h. iv
Klebsiella	Aminoglycoside	
	+	
	Cephalosporin	
	Cefoxitin	3 g q.4h. iv
	Cefamandole	3 g q.4h. iv
Serratia	Aminoglycoside	
	Cephalosporin	
	Ticarcillin	
	Carbenicillin	
Enterobacter	Gentamicin	
	Tobramycin	
Escherichia coli	Aminoglycoside	
	Cephalosporin	
	Ampicillin	1 g q.4h. iv
Proteus mirabilis	Ampicillin	
	Ticarcillin	
	Carbenicillin	
	Cephalosporin	

well-aerated tissues where sporangia germinate from inhaled spores. The vegetative forms have broad nonseptate hyphae with right-angled branching. In rhinocerebral mucormycosis, the fungus invades through the palatal, nasal, or paranasal sinus mucosa, ultimately reaching the brain.

A *Rhizopus oryzae* palatal lesion with a greenish-white center and black margins in a child undergoing treatment for acute lymphocytic leukemia is shown in figure 4–16**B**. The hyphae penetrated into the underlying tissue and walls of the local blood vessels leading to angitis, thrombosis, and ischemic necrosis. The infection subsequently extended into the ethmoid sinus, face, orbit, meninges, and frontal lobe of the brain before the patient expired. As with aspergillosis, mucormycosis is almost invariably fatal unless the cancer is brought into remission and adequate therapy with amphotericin B is provided.

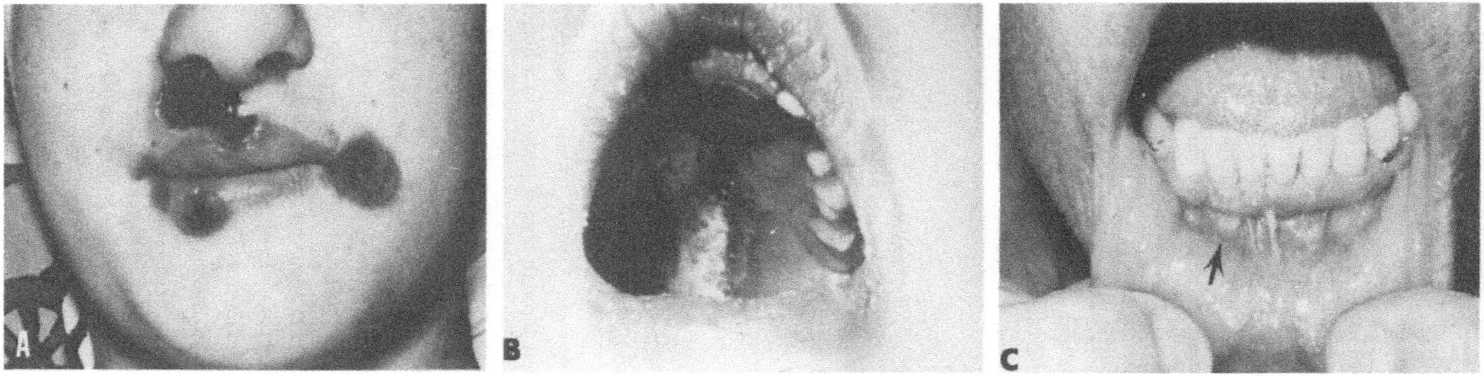

Figure 4–16. Noncandidal oral fungal infections in patients undergoing cancer chemotherapy.

A. Intraoral and circumoral *A. fumigatus* infection in patient with acute myelogenous leukemia.

B. Palatal *R. oryzae* infection in patient with acute lymphocytic leukemia.

C. Gingival histoplasmosis in patient with Hodgkin's lymphoma.

Histoplasmosis

Most histoplasmosis infections in immunosuppressed patients, particularly those with leukemia or lymphoma, seem to be due to recent exposure to the fungus rather than to an exacerbation of prior healed pulmonary disease [24]. Although histoplasmosis is usually manifested as a generalized disease that most often affects the lungs or reticuloendothelial system, localized lesions may occur in the absence of systemic involvement. *Histoplasma capsulatum,* a small oval yeast-like organism that shows budding on culture, apparently enters the body in spore form through the mouth or nose where the organism may germinate to produce focal lesions. Clinically, these range from wart-like papillary tumors represented by the gingival lesion in a patient receiving chemotherapy for Hodgkin's lymphoma (figure 4–16**C**) to nodules, vegetations, and ulcerations in the lips, tongue, and palate that grossly simulate tuberculosis. The preferred antifungal agent for the treatment of histoplasmosis is amphotericin B.

Bacterial infections

Gram-negative bacillary infections

The pattern of life-threatening bacterial infections in patients immunocompromised by cancer chemotherapy has changed drastically since the advent of the broad-spectrum antibiotics and penicillinase-resistant penicillins. Gram-positive coccal infections in the chemotherapy patient have been surpassed by gram-negative bacillary infections in frequency and severity. These organisms are seldom pathogenic in individuals with intact host defenses and their prevalence in the oropharyngeal bacterial flora of a healthy population is extremely low [13]. The vast majority of the oral gram-negative bacillary infections in cancer patients are associated with chemotherapy-induced immunosuppression that depletes both the systemic and local-tissue barriers to infection. They stem from exposure of the drug and disease debilitated patient to species of *Pseudomonas, Klebsiella, Serratia, Enterobacter, Proteus,* and *Escherichia* made increasingly virulent through human passage in a hospital setting.

Pseudomonas infections

Pseudomonas species can survive in hospitals for long periods of time since they are highly resistant to the usual methods of asepsis. This organism is so nonfastidious in nutritional needs that it requires none of the usual growth factors and can utilize atmospheric carbon dioxide as a sole source of carbon and ammonium as a sole source of nitrogen. As evidenced by stool and throat cultures, more than half the patients with acute leukemia become carriers of *Pseudomonas* within the first four weeks of hospitalization [12]. Both the nonpigmented and pyocin-typable strains are capable of producing mouth infections in patients subjected to cancer chemotherapy.

Almost all of the *Pseudomonas* lesions are caused by *P. aeruginosa.* This species has a faculty for producing necrotizing proteolytic enzymes, for invading the walls of small arteries and veins to produce vasculitis, and for repelling leukocytes. The oral lesions may involve the lips (figure 4–17**A**), gingiva (figure 4–17**B**), palate, tongue, and palatine tonsils.

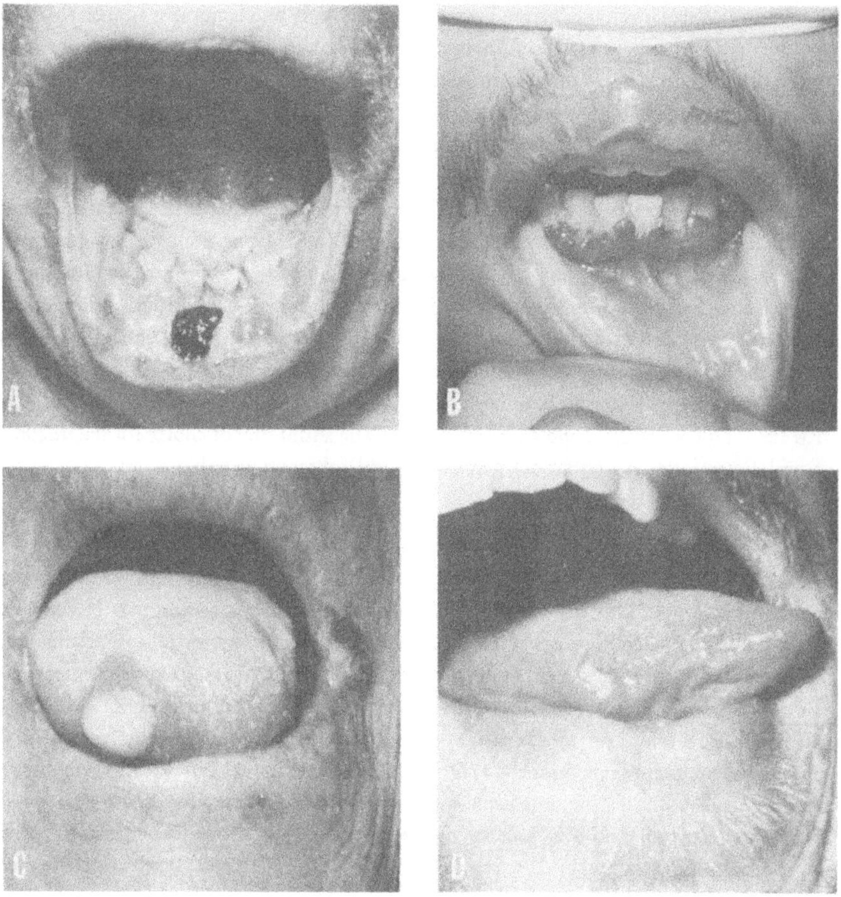

Figure 4–17. Oral gram-negative bacillary infections in patients receiving cancer chemotherapy.

A. *P. aeruginosa* infection of inside of lip in patient with blastic phase of chronic myelogenous leukemia.
B. *P. aeruginosa* infection in gingiva of patient with acute myelogenous leukemia.
C. *E. cloacae* infection in tongue and lips of patient in blastic phase of chronic myelogenous leukemia.
D. *E. coli* infection of tongue in patient with acute myelogenous leukemia.

They are featured by a purple to black necrotic center encircled by a narrow red halo. There is a conspicuous lack of leukocyte response evidenced by the absence of a visible exudate. With time, the necrotic area becomes sharply demarcated from the surrounding uninvolved tissue and sloughs en masse leaving a glistening, raw-red base of viable granulation tissue. As listed in table 4–5, the most efficacious treatment for oral *Pseudomonas* infections is ticarcillin or carbenicillin alone or in combination with an aminoglycoside like gentamicin, tobramycin, or amikacin.

Enterobacter infections

Enterobacter (Aerobacter) species are bacteriologically and biochemically similar to *E. coli* and even more closely related to *K. pneumoniae.* Although usually considered more saprophytic than either of these organisms, *Enterobacter* species have contributed to the general increase in nosocomial infections caused by indigenous gram-negative bacilli in medically compromised patients. Despite the reputedly low pathogenicity of *Enterobacter,* almost half of the oral infections produced by this species in cancer patients have been monoinfections.

Enterobacter-precipitated oral infections have presented as peritonsillar abscesses, glossitis, and cheilitis. An *E. cloacae* infection that produced focal, penetrating yellow-pigmented colonization on the tongue and left commissure of the lips in a patient treated for chronic myelogenous leukemia in the blastic phase is shown in figure 4–17**C**. Mouth lesions created by *E. aerogenes* are porcelain-white, moist, patchy, elevated, and conglomerate. They are extremely painful, erosive, and productive of shallow ulcers. Mixed infections of the oral cavity involving *Enterobacter* have been manifested mainly as an ulceromembranous gingivitis affecting the marginal and attached gingiva. The antibiotics of choice for the treatment of oral *Enterobacter* infections are gentamicin and tobramycin (table 4–5).

Escherichia infections

E. coli is a leading cause of opportunistic gram-negative bacillary infections in both general and cancer hospitals. Like the other nosocomials, the offending organism may be a member of the patient's normal flora or be acquired after hospital admission. Disease results when the organism is introduced into an area where local host defenses are severely depressed.

Oral monoinfections with *E. coli* have been confined to the tongue, lips, and gingiva. The lesions are white-surfaced, erosive, exudative, edematous, and erythematous in the acute stage and as shown in figure 4–17**D**, ulcerative thereafter. *E. coli* has also been isolated from patients with mixed organisms gingivitis in association with *Klebsiella, Serratia, Enterobacter, Proteus,* and *Pseudomonas* either singly or in various combinations. Mouth infections by *E. coli* are usually sensitive to the aminoglycosides, cephalosporins, and broad-spectrum penicillins (table 4–5).

Klebsiella infections

In the past decade there has been a notable increase in the incidence of *Klebsiella* infections and superinfections in patients undergoing cancer chemotherapy. *K. pneumoniae,* an encapsulated gram-negative rod, has been identified as an opportunistic pathogen in up to 10% of acquired infections in hospitalized cancer patients. Antibiotic therapy predisposing to intestinal colonization of *Klebsiella* has been implicated as a reservoir of the organism [25]. Virulence as measured by bacteremia and mortality has not been confined to a particular capsular type of strain. Adding to the intensity of the problem in cancer patients is the recent emergence of strains resistant to most antibiotics [26].

The intraoral lesions produced by *K. pneumoniae* (figure 4–18**A**) are creamy white, raised, glistening, spreading, and superficially erosive on a reddened base. They are painful, nonpurulent, and often covered with an adherent grayish-white pseudomembrane. Lesions may develop in any part of the mouth or pharynx but occur mainly on the tongue, gingiva,

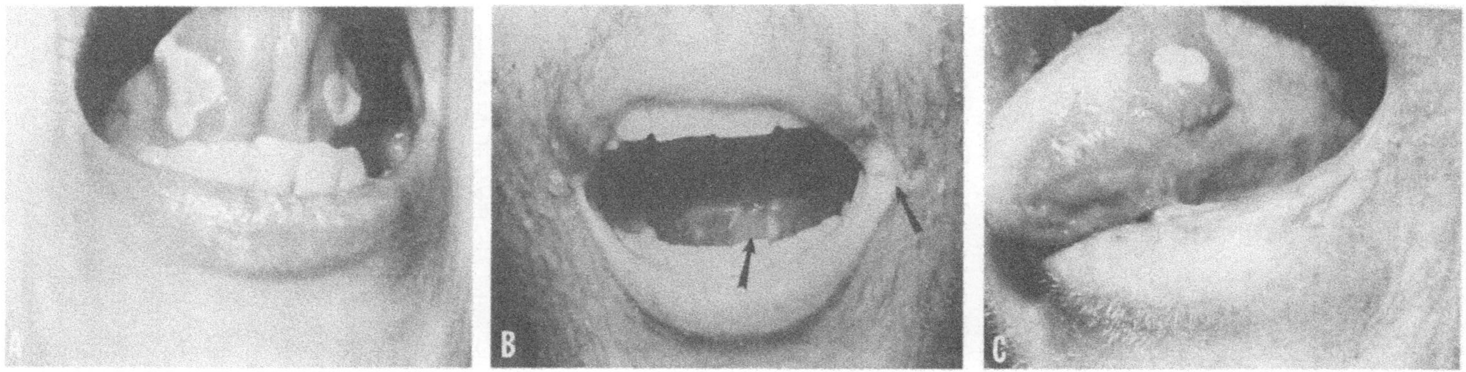

Figure 4–18. Oral gram-negative bacillary infections in patients receiving cancer chemotherapy.

A. *K. pneumoniae* infection of undersurface of tongue in patient with acute myelogenous leukemia.
B. *S. marcescens* infection in tongue and lips of patient with acute myelogenous leukemia.
C. *P. mirabilis* infection in tongue of patient with acute myelogenous leukemia.

lips, and palate. Oral *K. pneumoniae* infections respond best to a combination of an aminoglycoside and a cephalosporin-like cefoxitin and cefamandole (table 4–5).

Serratia infections

Infections attributable to *Serratia* (especially *S. marcescens*), long considered a harmless saprophyte, are being diagnosed with increasing frequency in patients hospitalized for cancer chemotherapy. Most have occurred subsequent to exposure to broad-spectrum antibiotics and have taken the form of septicemia, pneumonitis, pyelonephritis, osteomyelitis, skin ulcers, and stomatitis. *S. marcescens* thrives in a moist environment and lives in hospital equipment. Some strains produce a pink pigment (prodigiosin) when grown in the dark. The vast majority of strains recovered from human infections, however, have been nonchromogenic.

A *S. marcescens* glossitis and cheilitis that developed in a patient during treatment for acute myelogenous leukemia is shown in figure 4–18**B**. *Serratia* induced oral lesions usually consist of very painful ulcers with marginal white colonization. They often arise at sites of tissue-trauma-like denture sores. *Serratia* frequently produces superinfections in oral lesions initiated by other organisms. In such instances the morphologic characteristics of the lesions are altered to that of shallow erosions covered by an off-white pseudomembrane teeming with microbes. Amikacin and gentamicin are the most active antibiotics against *Serratia.* Some strains are sensitive to carbenicillin and ticarcillin, others to the cephalosporins (table 4–5).

Proteus infections

Almost all of the oral *Proteus* infections in the cancer chemotherapy population are caused by *P. mirabilis.* This is the only indole-negative species of a genus that historically has been mainly associated with urinary tract infections. The typical swarming pattern of *Proteus* when grown on agar is duplicated in large part on the mucosal and skin surfaces of infected patients.

A *P. mirabilis* infection that covered almost the entire two-thirds of the dorsum and produced a painful abscess surrounded by a zone of erythema at the left margin of the tongue in a patient with acute myelogenous leukemia is shown in figure 4–18**C**. The lingual colonization was slightly raised, mildly erosive, glistening, adherent, yellow-tinged, and wavy in appearance. *Proteus* has also been a common contributor to mixed-organism gingivitis in immunosuppressed cancer patients. The most useful antibiotics against *P. mirabilis* are ampicillin, carbenicillin, ticarcillin, and the cephalosporins (table 4–5).

Except for those produced by *Pseudomonas,* the oral lesions caused by pure and mixed gram-negative bacillary infections are clinically indistinguishable. All are essentially similar in appearance, course, and distribution. They are differentiated from one another only by direct culture of the lesion and bacteriologic identification of the organism. No single antibiotic has been effective against all strains of gram-negative bacilli recovered from oral lesions of cancer patients. Broad-spectrum antibiotics in the form of a combination of a semisynthetic penicillin (ticarcillin or carbenicillin) and an aminoglycoside (gentamicin or tobramycin) or a combination of a semisynthetic penicillin and cephalothin should be administered immediately following the appearance of an oral lesion to minimize the danger of gram-negative sepsis. The antibiotic coverage should be continued until antibiotic sensitivity tests of isolates from the lesion permit strain-specific treatment.

Gram-positive coccal infections

Staphylococcal infections

Both *S. aureus* and *S. epidermidis* are ubiquitous human parasites that are part of the normal nasal and skin flora. They are differentiated on the basis of colony color on blood agar and ability to produce coagulase. The golden-yellow *S. aureus* is coagulase-positive; the white *S. epidermidis,* coagulase-negative. Although each species is extremely pyogenic giving rise to purulent lesions in patients with normal granulocyte counts, oral mucosal lesions produced by these organisms in granulocytopenic cancer patients are dry, plaque-like, verrucous, and white to dark brown in color.

S. aureus infections of the dorsum of the tongue that developed during treatment for acute myelogenous leukemia and of the lips and palatal mucosa that emerged during treatment for adenocarcinoma of the lung are shown in figures 4–19**A** and 4–19**B**. *S. epidermidis* lip lesions in patients receiving chemotherapy for histiocytic lymphoma and for acute myelogenous leukemia are shown in figures 4–19**C** and 4–19**D**. *S. aureus* infections of the mouth are responsive to penicillinase-resistant antibiotics like methicillin, whereas *S. epidermidis* may be sensitive to penicillin G. Some recently recovered strains of *S. epidermidis* have been insensitive to most antibiotics, responding only to vancomycin and rifampin (table 4–5).

Streptococcal infections

The great preponderance of documented oral streptococcal infections in patients subjected to the antineoplastic drugs are caused by either *S. faecalis* or *S. pyogenes.* Both the group D variably hemolytic enterococcus, *S. faecalis,* and the group A hemolytic *S. pyogenes* may be present in healthy mouths. Oral enterococcal infections associated with cancer chemotherapy take the form of white to grayish-white colonization of the labial, gingival, lingual, and palatal mucosa. The organism is a common secondary infector of herpetic lip ulcers in such patients. *S. pyogenes* has been isolated from the grayish-white exudate of chemotherapy precipitated acute tonsillitis and from the mixed flora in cancer patients with operculitis involving partially erupted third molars. The antibiotics of choice for oral enterococcal infections is a combination of penicillin G and gentamicin; for *S. pyogenes* infections, penicillin G alone (table 4–5).

Viral infections

Herpes simplex infections

Although many of the antitumor drugs inhibit DNA synthesis, Herpes simplex (a DNA virus) is frequently activated in the lips of patients harboring the virus during cancer chemotherapy. Onset of the infection is signaled by tautness, itching, and burning of the lips followed by the emergence of papulovesicles that rupture, ulcerate, and become

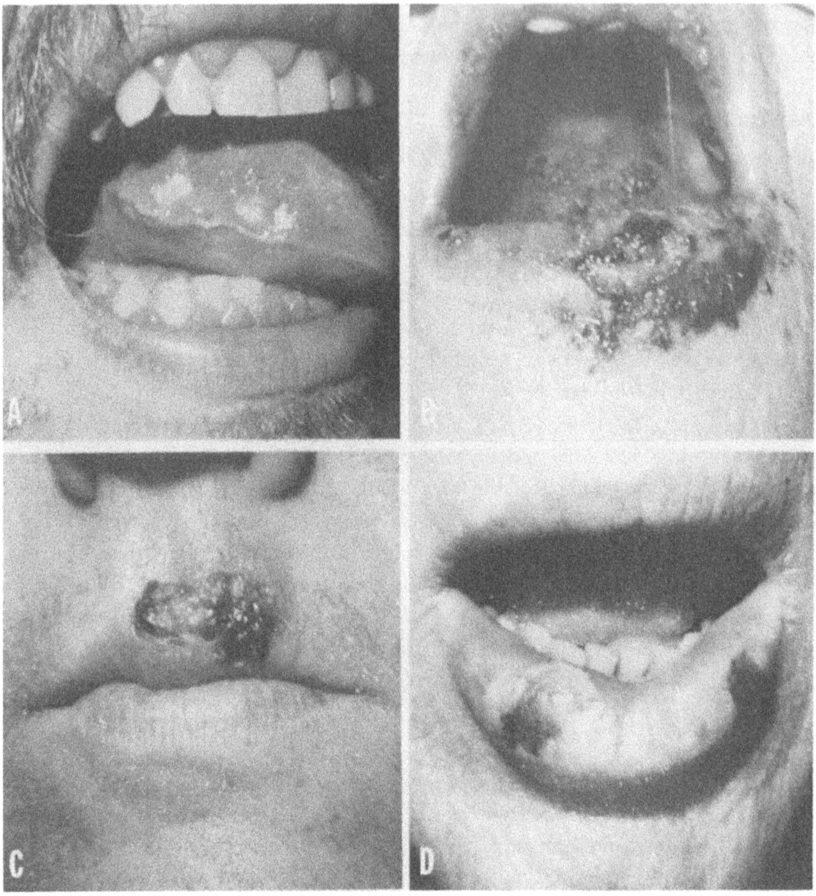

Figure 4–19. Oral staphylococcal infections in patients receiving cancer chemotherapy.

A. *S. aureus* infection on dorsum of tongue in patient with acute myelogenous leukemia.
B. *S. aureus* infection of lips and palate in patient with adenocarcinoma of lung.
C. *S. epidermidis* infection in lip of patient with diffuse histiocytic lymphoma.
D. *S. epidermidis* infection in lip of patient with acute myelogenous leukemia.

encrusted. Often they cover large areas of the labial mucosa and cross the vermillion border onto the circumoral skin (figure 4–20**A**). Many become superinfected with *Candida* (figures 4–20**B** and 4–20**C**) and/or bacteria. Some develop into herpes phagedena manifested by large, chronic, encrusted ulcers that last weeks or months before resolving.

In rare instances the infection may spread to the mouth, pharynx, esophagus, lung, and brain. In most cases the lip lesions regress uneventfully in 10 to 14 days. There is no antiviral agent that is totally effective against all oral herpes infections. Some amelioration has been obtained by frequent topical applications of either 0.05% idoxuridine in a petrolatum-base ointment or 3% vidarabine in a mixture of solid and liquid petrolatum (table 4–5).

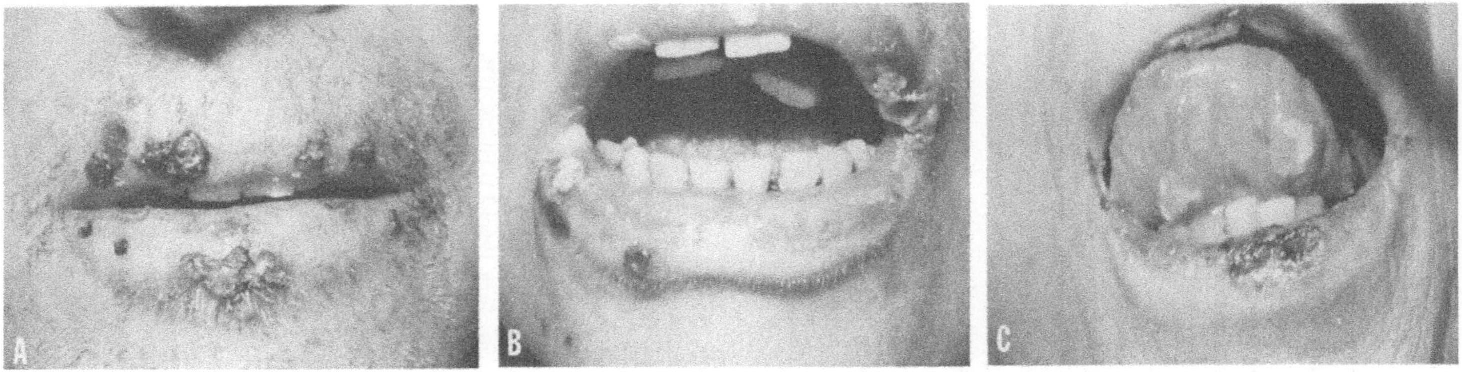

Figure 4–20. Oral herpetic infections in patients undergoing cancer chemotherapy.

A. Herpes simplex infection of lips and circumoral skin in patient with adenocarcinoma of colon.
B. Herpes labialis and lingual candidiasis in patient with adenocarcinoma of ampulla.
C. Herpes labialis and labial candidiasis in patient with acute myelogenous leukemia.

Other viral infections

Like Herpes simplex virus, the varicella-zoster and cytomegaloviruses are uniquely able to attack susceptible hosts and are opportunistic agents par excellence. A progressive varicella that may produce pustular lesions on the tongue and oral mucosa occurs fairly frequently in children with leukemia. Both radiation therapy and chemotherapy have been associated with the development of zoster in patients with malignant disease. The typical skin lesions heralded by radicular pain usually present as a unilateral eruption encompassing from one to three dermatomes. Except for the ophthalmic division of the trigeminal nerve, zoster rarely affects the cranial nerves to the face and mouth in the chemotherapy patient. Similarly, save for parotitis, cytomegalovirus infection of the oral structures is extremely uncommon even in debilitated immunosuppressed cancer patients with cytomegalovirus pneumonitis, hepatitis, and other signs of disseminated disease.

In summary, the immunosuppressive, myelosuppressive, and cytotoxic effects of cancer chemotherapy deprive the patient of almost all natural defenses against microbial infection. Every oral infection in such patients constitutes a major threat to well-being and survival. None should be dismissed summarily as of no consequence. There are no benign oral infections in patients lacking protection against microbial attack. Each must be treated vigorously and brought under control as quickly as possible to prevent potentially fatal consequences.

REFERENCES

1. Goodman LS, Wintrobe MM, Dameshek W. Goodman MJ, Gilman A, McLennan MT: Nitrogen mustard therapy: Use of methyl-bis (β-chloroethyl) amine hydrochloride and tris (β-chloroethyl) amine hydrochloride for Hodgkin's disease, lymphosarcoma, leukemia and certain allied and miscellaneous disorders. J AMA 132:126–132, 1946.
2. Rauscher FJ Jr: National Cancer Program. Report of the Director. DHEW Publication No. (NIH) 77–472, 1977.
3. Bodey GP, Hersh EM, Valdivieso M, Feld R, Rodriguez V: Effects of cytotoxic and immunosuppressive agents on the immune system. Postgrad Med 58:67–74, 1975.
4. Levine AS, Schimpff SC, Grow RG Jr, Young RC: Hematologic malignancies and other marrow failure states: Progress in the management of complicating infections. Semin Hematol 11:141–202, 1974.
5. Bodey GP, Buckley M, Sathe YS, Freireich EJ: Quantitative relationships between circulating leukocytes and infection in patients with acute leukemia. Ann Intern Med 64:328–340, 1966.
6. Strumia MM, Boerner F: Phagocytic activity of circulating cells in the various types of leukemia. Am J Pathol 13:335–349, 1937.
7. Dreizen, S, Bodey GP, Rodriguez V: Oral complications of cancer chemotherapy. Postgrad Med 58:75–82, 1975.
8. Dreizen S, McCredie KB, Keating MJ: Chemotherapy-induced oral mucositis in adult leukemia. Postgrad Med 69:103–112, 1981.
9. Lockhart PB, Sonis ST: Relationship of oral complications to peripheral blood leukocyte and platelet counts in patients receiving cancer chemotherapy. Oral Surg 48:21–28, 1979.
10. Schimpff SC: Infections in the compromised host. In *Principles and Practice of Infectious Diseases.* Mandell GL, Douglass RG, Bennett JE (eds), New York, John Wiley & Sons 1979, pp 2257–2262.
11. Schimpff SC, Young VM, Greene WH, Vermeulen GD, Moody MR, Wiernik PH: Origin of infection in acute nonlymphocytic leukemia. Ann Intern Med 77:707–714, 1972.
12. Bodey GP: Epidemiological studies of *Pseudomonas* species in patients with leukemia. Am J Med Sci 260:82–89, 1970.
13. Johanson WG, Pierce AK, Stanford JP: Changing pharyngeal bacterial flora of hospitalized patients. Emergence of gram negative bacilli. N Engl J Med 251:1137–1140, 1969.
14. Dreizen S, McCredie KB, Bodey GP: Unusual mucocutaneous infections in immunosuppressed patients with leukemia. Postgrad Med 66:131–141, 1979.

15. Lavelle CLB: Prevention of oral infections in patients receiving cancer therapy. J Can Dent Assn 42:551–553, 1976.
16. Dreizen S, McCredie KB, Keating MJ, Bodey GP: Chemotherapy-associated oral infection in adults with acute leukemia. Postgrad Med 71:133–146, 1982.
17. Dreizen S, Bodey GP, Validivieso M: Chemotherapy-associated oral infections in patients with solid tumors (in preparation).
18. DeVita VT, Young RC: Infection and cancer: Old friends. Ann Intern Med 79:579–599, 1973.
19. Brown LR, Dreizen S, Bodey GP: Effect of immunosuppression on the human oral flora. In *Comparative Immunology of the Oral Cavity,* Mergenhagen SE, Scherp HW (eds), Bethesda, Md DHEW Publication No. (NIH) 73–438, 1973 pp 204–220.
20. Brown LR, Dreizen S, Horton IM, Steacy E, Perkins D, Wheatcroft MG, Bodey GP, McCredie KB: Cultivable plaque microflora of cancer patients treated in conventional and protected environments. J Dent Res 58:338, 1979 (Special Issue A).
21. Wheatcroft M, Dreizen S, Steacy E, Brown L, Bodey G, McCredie K: Cinemicrographic profiles of plaque microflora of cancer patients treated in protective and conventional environments. J Dent Res 58:338, 1979 (Special Issue A).
22. Bodey GP: Infectious complications of acute leukemia. Med Times 94:1076–1085, 1966.
23. Schimpff SC: Infections in patients with acute leukemia. In *Principles and Practice of Infectious Diseases.* Mandell GL, Douglass RG, Bennett JE (eds), New York, John Wiley & Sons, 1979, pp 2263–2278.
24. Kauffman CA, Israel KS, Smith JW, White AC, Schwarz J, Brooks GF: Histoplasmosis in immunosuppressed patients. Am J Med 64:923–932, 1978.
25. Selden R, Lee S, Wang WLL, Bennett JV, Eickhoff TC: Nosocomial klebsiella infections: Intestinal colonization as a reservoir. Ann Intern Med 74:657–664, 1971.
26. Bodey GP: Infections in cancer patients. Cancer Treat Rev 2:89–128, 1975.

5. BACTERIAL INFECTIONS: PERIODONTAL AND DENTAL DISEASE

DOUGLAS E. PETERSON, D.M.D., Ph.D.

INTRODUCTION

Infections in the myelosuppressed cancer patient are serious sequelae of both the natural disease as well as the chemotherapy used in its treatment. For example, infection is the leading cause of morbidity and mortality in patients with acute nonlymphocytic leukemia (ANLL) [1,2]. Prevention, recognition, and treatment of acute infections in the cancer patient receiving chemotherapy are critical to his/her quality and duration of life.

The role of periodontal and dental infections in the cancer patient receiving myelosuppressive chemotherapy has not always been recognized; it is only recently that the frequency and severity have been adequately understood. Historically, many clinicians have categorized most oral complications as mucositis. One should note that both mucositis and infections involving the periodontium are types of stomatitis [3–14]; this distinction is important since the pathogenesis of each of the two lesions is uniquely different. In addition, most pulpal complications, again distinct from mucositis, result from the exacerbation of periapical infection present prior to myelosuppression; in our experience, periapical disease newly developed during the period of profound granulocytopenia is not frequent.

The distinction between the processes of mucositis, periodontal, and pulpal disease is critical for the proper management of cancer patients. Unless close cooperation exists between the medical, dental, and nursing staffs, these patients may not receive adequate pretreatment oral evaluation, and much of the chronic infection resident within the oral cavity might not be properly diagnosed. Only through interdisciplinary communication

D.E. Peterson and S.T. Sonis (eds.), ORAL COMPLICATIONS OF CANCER CHEMOTHERAPY, 79-91.

can comprehensive oral management of the patient be achieved. This chapter will address periodontal and dental pulpal complications (including their recognition and treatment as well as, ideally, their prevention) in the patient undergoing myelosuppressive chemotherapy. Much of this discussion will focus upon patients with ANLL since this population often develops these complications.

ANATOMY

A clear understanding of the periodontal and pulpal structures is essential to appreciation of related complications that arise. The periodontium is the supporting and nutritive apparatus of the dentition and includes the gingiva, alveolar bone, periodontal ligament, and cementum. Under healthy conditions, the space between the nonkeratinized sulcular epithelium and the cementum does not exceed three mm in depth, as measured by a calibrated periodontal probe. The microbial flora of this normal environment is primarily aerobic in the supragingival plaque (facultative cocci, bacilli, and fusobacteria) and anaerobic in the subgingival plaque (anaerobic rods and cocci) [15,16].

Periodontal disease (figure 5–1) reflects an inflammatory response to bacteria that colonize the surface of the tooth contiguous to the gingiva, metabolize local nutrients, and elaborate toxins which eventually penetrate the epithelium of the gingival sulcus. As in patients without periodontal disease, subgingival plaque is constitutionally different from supragingival plaque; the subgingival plaque is primarily gram-negative and anaerobic (motile rods, vibrios, and spirochetes).

Thus the disease can be characterized as an inflammatory response to metabolites of a mixed infection established on the tooth surface. The earliest, most obvious clinical symptom of periodontal disease in patients without cancer is bleeding, representing an ulcerated epithelial surface. In the patient with severe periodontal disease, the total surface area of the ulceration can easily exceed two cm^2; even with this extensive lesion, the patient is often unaware of any oral pathology. The extent of disease can only be detected by clinical and radiographic examination.

Contrasted with the periodontium is the dental pulp, which normally represents the vital component of the tooth itself and consists of vascular, nervous, cellular, lymphatic, and collagenous elements within a ground substance (figure 5–2). Its chief role occurs during dentin formation; after dentinogenesis is complete, the pulp gradually diminishes in volume throughout the life of the patient. It is capable of transmitting thermal and pain sensations.

Irreversible injury to the dental pulp (caused by physical, chemical, or bacterial factors) can lead to acute pulpitis and/or pulpal necrosis. Depending upon the nature of injury involved, an infection of the periapical tissue may develop. One such predominant cause of pulpal insult is dental caries, which is a bacterial infection. Thus it is not unusual that infectious complications in myelosuppressed cancer patients may develop secondary to such commonly observed pathology as dental caries.

ACUTE PERIODONTAL INFECTION IN PATIENTS RECEIVING CHEMOTHERAPY

Even in patients without cancer, periodontal disease is very common; up to 98% of the adult population in the United States has some degree of involvement [17]. It similarly occurs in patients newly admitted for intensive chemotherapy (table 5–1; figure 5–1). As

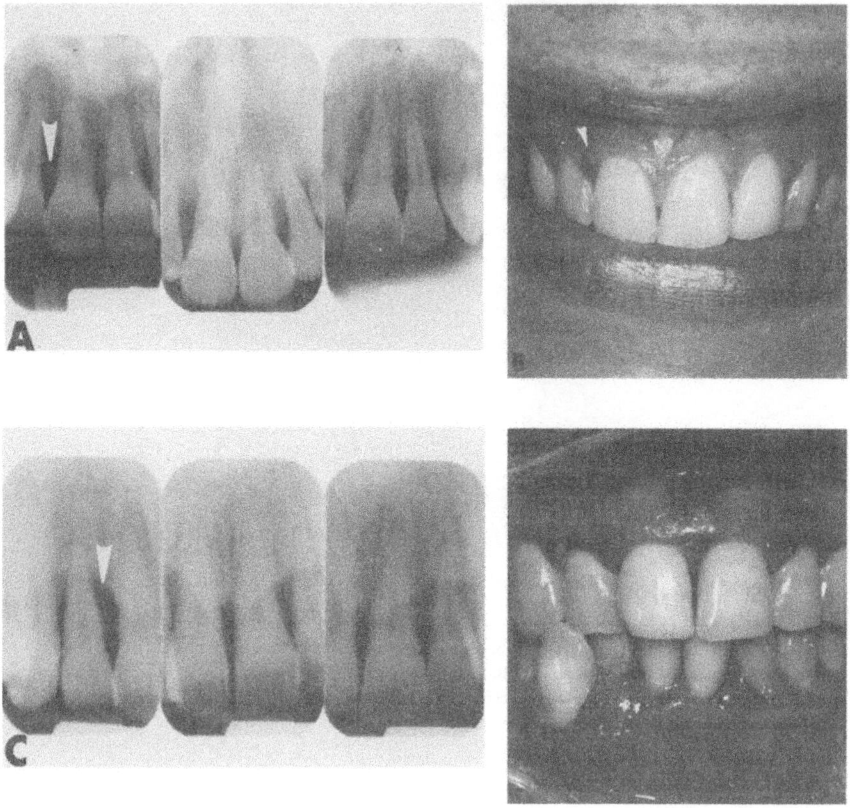

Figure 5–1. Periodontitis.

A. Radiograph demonstrates bony dissolution *(arrow)* as can appear in patient with moderate periodontitis. Periodontal probing revealed 4-mm pocket depth in this area.

B. Clinical appearance reveals subtle evidence of an acute exacerbation of moderate periodontitis in this acute nonlymphocytic leukemic patient with granulocyte level $<100/\mu l$. Ulcerative nature of periodontal pocket is not clinically evident. Patient described intense pain in the maxillary anterior *(arrow)* and was febrile.

C. Extensive loss of bone as viewed on radiograph *(arrow)* in a patient with severe periodontitis. The two maxillary incisors exhibited marked mobility. Periodontal pocket depth measured 7 mm.

D. Clinical appearance of severe periodontitis. The granulocyte level in this acute nonlymphocytic patient was $>1000/\mu l$. Again the extensive ulceration of this lesion is not directly observed. This patient, however, did not develop a periodontal exacerbation during subsequent chemotherapy.

(Source: Reprinted with permission from Arch Intern Med 142:551–554, 1982. Copyright 1982, American Medical Association.)

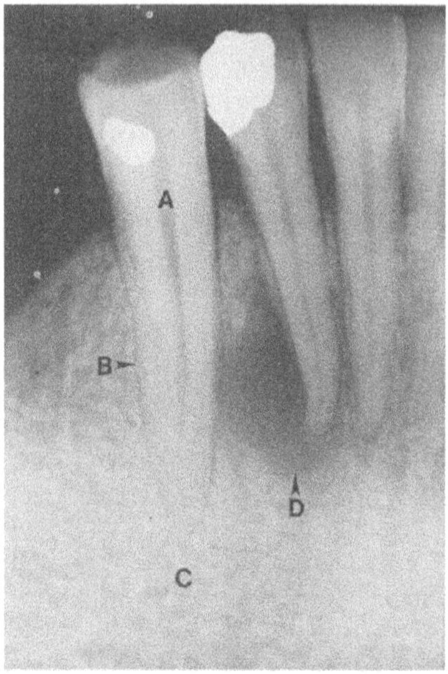

Figure 5–2. Dental Pulp. Radiograph demonstrates both healthy and diseased periapical tissue. Note normal-appearing dental pulp **(A)**, periodontal ligament space **(B)**, and alveolar bone **(C)**. This patient had an acute infection periapical to the lateral incisor **(D)**, secondary to a necrotic pulp. This lesion was present in a newly diagnosed, febrile (38.3°C) acute myelogenous leukemia patient with no other obvious source of infection.

(Radiograph courtesy Dr. E.J. Hovland.)

in most patients with this chronic infection, the process is usually asymptomatic and the cancer patient is often unaware of its presence or severity. The acute complications associated with periodontal disease arise during myelosuppression since, as noted earlier, the lesion is an ulcerative process. The following case describes such an episode of acute exacerbation of preexistent periodontal disease, which was successfully managed.

Table 5–1. Admitting periodontal status of patients with acute nonlymphocytic leukemia

	Number of Patients
Healthy periodontium	0
Gingivitis only	1
Moderate periodontal disease	17
Severe periodontal disease	21
Total number of patients	39

Case history

A 31-year-old white female with acute myelogenous leukemia was admitted for remission induction. Prior to such therapy, she was examined clinically and radiographically by the dental staff; moderate periodontal disease confined to the maxillary and mandibular premolar and molar regions, and three minor carious lesions were diagnosed. This patient had fair oral hygiene and was instructed to continue toothbrushing and flossing under the supervision of the dental hygienist.

The next day the patient was started on daunorubicin (45 mg/m^2 daily $\times$ three days) and cytosine arabinoside (100 mg/m^2 daily $\times$ seven days) as a continuous infusion. By the twelfth day, the patient's granulocyte count was $<100/\mu l$, platelets $30{,}000/\mu l$, and hematocrit 30%. On this day, she began to describe a mild soreness in the mandibular right molar region; the periodontium in this site was tender to palpation and she was febrile (38.4°C).

The next day, the discomfort became more severe, and her temperature rose to 39.0°C. Local home care (toothbrushing, flossing) was reinforced, and irrigation with topical peroxide was instituted; broad-spectrum systemic antibiotic therapy was initiated. No other sites of acute infection were clinically documented; no bacteremias were detected.

Twenty-four hours later, the oral complaint had mitigated, and the temperature was 37.2°C. By the following day, no oral symptoms were noted; temperature was normal.

Exacerbations such as just described are extremely prevalent [18–25], accounting for up to 28% of all acute infections in patients with ANLL [25]. The ulceration can be a direct portal of entry for the oral microflora; *Klebsiella pneumoniae, Enterobacter aerogenes,* and *Staphylococcal epidermidis* are organisms that can easily penetrate this ulcerated lesion, resulting in septicemia [24]. However, further study is needed to document which organisms might be involved in the acute infections which, if treated promptly, do not usually result in bacteremia.

It has been demonstrated that 47% of all acute infections in the myelosuppressed leukemic patient are caused by organisms acquired within the hospital [1]. Disease and debilitation can cause shifts in oral microbial flora [26,27], as can chemotherapy-induced myelosuppression; for example, gram-negative bacilli and *Candida spp.* become predominant in the mouths of acute leukemia patients undergoing induction [28,29]. However, most oral cultures, including surveillance cultures [30], do not usually assay the subgingival flora; this flora presumably includes the etiologic agents of acute periodontal infection during myelosuppression. Thus a study that assesses both the shifts in the subgingival flora as well as the microorganisms causative for the acute infections is critical. Such a study is presently ongoing at the University of Maryland Cancer Center (UMCC). To date, preliminary data from 20 patients suggest that many acute periodontal exacerbations are not caused by some of the major pathogens associated with mortality in ANLL *(Proteus spp., Escherichia coli, Aspergillus spp., Pseudomonas spp.)* [1,2]. It also appears that a quantitative, but not qualitative, shift occurs in the microbial population during prolonged, profound granulocytopenia. Further study is required to elaborate these preliminary findings. One should note that techniques used in such a study are tedious and specialized. As stated previously, the subgingival flora are usually gram-negative anaerobes, which require careful laboratory technique to maintain viability. Accurate identification is not likely if these organisms are not properly cultured.

Naturally, it would be ideal to prevent the acute periodontal infection from occurring initially. Views on the best approach to this goal have varied substantially, with some oncologists advocating full-mouth extractions in patients in leukemic remission [31], and others recommending avoiding any oral-hygiene care during induction, which often extends into several weeks' duration. Great concern regarding the effect of bacteremias established secondary to oral tissue manipulation still exists in the minds of many oncologists. This clinical dilemma has evolved because of the lack of care coordinated between the oncologist, the dentist, and the nurse.

At the UMCC, we are conducting a prospective, randomized trial of ANLL patients to determine the proper oral care of the periodontium during induction. To date, 19 patients have received limited oral hygiene care (consisting of toothbrushing and flossing instructions only) and 20 have received thorough oral hygiene care (similar instructions and supervision, plus an intensive dental scaling prior to initiation of chemotherapy). Dental flossing is being used because of its effective, safe nature when performed properly [32,33]. Days of granulocytopenia (500–999/μl, 100–499/μl, and $<100/\mu$l), and compliance with nonabsorbable oral antibiotics have been comparable between the two groups.

Forty-five acute infections, documented as described previously [34], have occurred during myelosuppression in the 33 patients without diabetes and/or asymptomatic gingival leukemic infiltrate. Six of the 45 infections have been acute exacerbations of preexistent periodontal disease; five-sixths occurred in the limited oral hygiene patients (table 5–2). No increase in local or systemic complications (pharyngeal, esophageal, or pulmonary tracts) has been noted in the thorough oral hygiene group; all patients in this group whose granulocyte level $<2{,}000/\mu$l received prophylactic antibiotic coverage prior to scaling and polishing.* As with nonperiodontal infections [35,36], most acute infections involving the periodontium have occurred when the granulocyte count was markedly depressed ($<100/\mu$l). Patients with adult-onset diabetes mellitus and/or gingival leukemic infiltrate who received thorough oral hygiene care have developed acute periodontal exacerbations more

Table 5–2. Oral infections in acute nonlymphocytic leukemia patients without diabetes or asymptomatic gingival infiltrate at admission

	Limited hygiene	Thorough hygiene
Number of patients	18	15
Number of acute periodontal infections	5 (22%)[1]	1 (5%)
Number of acute oral, nonperiodontal infections	4 (18%)	4 (18%)
Total number of oral infections	9	5

[1]Number of infections/total number of infections in each patient group.

*Ticarcillin, Beecham Products, Briston, Tenn. 37620
Amikacin, Bristol Laboratories, Syracuse, N.Y. 13201

One-half hour before dental procedure:
Ticarcillin: 75 mg/kg by intravenous infusion
Amikacin: 4 mg/kg by intravenous infusion
Repeat regimen six hours after dental procedure.

frequently than thorough oral hygiene patients who did not have these underlying disorders.

It thus appears that rigorous attention to oral hygiene care can reduce the prevalence of a common oral complication of cancer chemotherapy. Proper supervision of the oral care must be stressed so that the patient does not injure the oral tissues. Since both groups of patients have had improved oral hygiene as measured by standardized indexes [37], it appears that the pretherapy dental scaling has played a vital role in reducing the prevalence of the complications. Quite possibly, the scaling might have initiated periodontal healing, promoted readaptation of the periodontium to the tooth, and thus reduced the portal of entry for the microbial flora.

In our experience most patients who develop acute periodontal infections respond well to local irrigation (10% carbamide peroxide) as well as broad-spectrum antibiotics (a penicillin-derivative plus an aminoglycoside) unlike some other infections described for this population [2,38]. However, each episode is a morbid event, causing considerable patient discomfort and requiring the use of local care and systemic antibiotics to resolve the acute phase.

It is also important to realize that bacteremias due to the oral hygiene care in this study did not result in adverse clinical sequelae. However, one would suspect that transient bacteremias did occur since such processes also occur in noncancer patients, with or without gingival disease [39–46]. We do not recommend the use of oral irrigation devices for myelosuppressed patients, due to extensive bacteremias that may develop [47]. We should remember that, even in a thrombocytopenic patient, gingival bleeding can indicate inflammation; spontaneous gingival bleeding usually occurs when platelet counts are $< 15{,}000/\mu l$. Failure to maintain excellent normal hygiene can result in increased bleeding compared to that seen with the proper use of oral hygiene aids, such as toothbrush and dental floss. Thus judicious use of toothbrush and floss can play a beneficial role in the oral supportive care of these patients.

This study has not demonstrated that improvement in oral hygiene resulted in lowered incidence of oral mucositis. This reduction has, however, been observed in previous studies [6,7,14]. We have found, however, that the ability to maintain overall good levels of oral hygiene was psychologically beneficial to the individuals on the protocol.

Cancer patients who present with acute infections prior to receiving chemotherapy require special attention; for example, acute leukemia patients acutely infected at admission have a lowered survival rate than those who are not acutely infected [48,49]. In a recent study, we reported that 89% of patients noninfected at admission achieved complete remission, compared to 58% patients who were infected at admission [50]. Acute periodontal infection, usually but not always in the form of leukemic infiltrate, accounted for 42% of all presenting infections. In such patients, levels of good oral hygiene are extremely difficult to achieve due to tumor infiltrate and gingival engorgement. In such patients, gentle toothbrushing, flossing, and swabbing with a moist gauze can improve oral hygiene; however, care must be taken (see chapter 7). Low-dose radiation (600 rad) of the gingiva may also be beneficial. Once induction is initiated, the gingival hyperplasia often partially resolves, lending the environment more accessible to hygiene care. Overall, however, this lesion is not easily managed and its presence indicates lessened chances for survival.

A detailed oral examination of every patient prior to chemotherapy should be performed. This examination should include diagnostic radiographs and use of the periodontal probe. Since the ulceration associated with periodontal disease cannot be directly visualized, these measures must be used to insure proper diagnosis.

Finally, periodontal therapy on a cancer patient in remission can be an effective means of improving the ability of the patient to maintain optimal periodontal health [51] (figure 5–3). On occasion, the cancer patient does not require re-treatment with antineoplastic agents for many months. This interval should be considered an opportunity to render the patient free of periodontal infection. Although dental extractions are one means by which this goal can be achieved, successful periodontal therapy can often achieve the same result and maintain the natural dentition. By eliminating periodontal disease, the risk for future acute periodontal infection during subsequent myelosuppressive episodes is markedly reduced.

DENTAL PULPAL DISEASE IN PATIENTS RECEIVING CHEMOTHERAPY

Although not extensively described in the literature, pulpal pathology can result in serious systemic infection [52,53]. In particular, infection arising from the dental pulp can contribute to the morbidity of the myelosuppressed cancer patient. This pathology, arising from

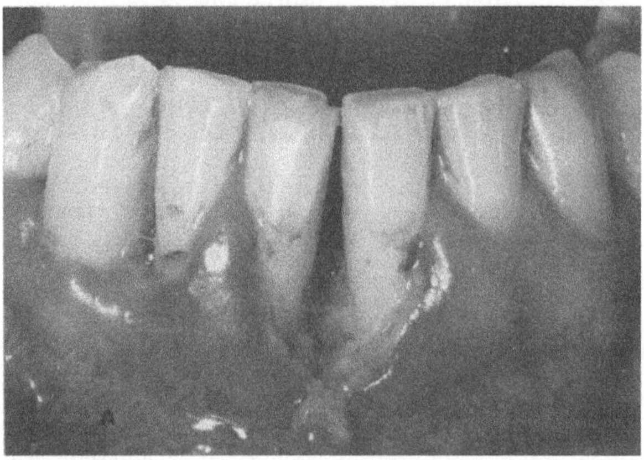

Figure 5–3. Periodontal Therapy

A. Acute periodontal infection between the mandibular central incisors in a patient receiving chemotherapy for metastatic breast carcinoma. The marked disruption in normal periodontal architecture rendered the site less amenable to optimal oral hygiene.

B. Smear of acute infection seen in figure 5–3**A**. *C. spp.* predominate, as evidenced by the hyphae. This patient was myelosuppressed and was experiencing acute pain.

C. The healthy appearance of the same region as figure 5–3**A** after periodontal therapy four months following cessation of chemotherapy. Note the interproximal regions accessible for the patient to maintain proper oral hygiene.

(Case and photographs courtesy Dr. J.B. Suzuki. Copyright by the American Dental Association. Reprinted by permission.)

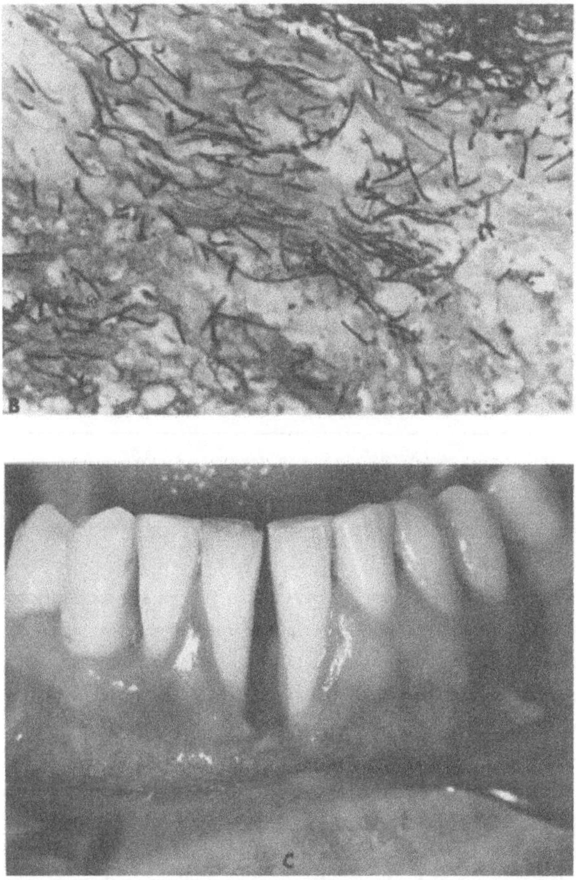

physical (mechanical, thermal, electrical), chemical, or bacterial injury, may result in irreversible pathology to the pulp. The pathology may or may not be symptomatic prior to onset of myelosuppression. As with periodontal disease, the oncologist should obtain a dental consult to rule out the presence of such a lesion, particularly of infectious nature, in any patient about to receive chemotherapy.

In patients whose functional granulocyte count is $> 1{,}000/\mu l$, specific signs and symptoms may be useful in determining whether the pulp has been irreversibly injured. If a patient describes spontaneous, throbbing pain, and/or pain brought on by hot or cold stimulus which lingers longer than fifteen seconds, one should suspect irreversible pulpal disease. Pain upon percussion is a result that usually indicates periapical disease secondary to irreversible pulpal disease. Radiographs, electric pulp, and thermal tests usually provide information sufficient for the diagnosis. In patients with functional granulocytes $< 1{,}000/\mu l$, percussion is not reliable and should not be used [21]. However, radiographs and thermal testing remain useful diagnostic aids.

The following case demonstrates that accurate diagnosis and prompt management can benefit the cancer patient receiving chemotherapy.

Case history

A 34-year-old white female was admitted with newly diagnosed acute myelogenous leukemia. Over the past two weeks, she had complained of mild fevers as well as spontaneous, sharp, lingering pain in the maxillary left premolar region during this time. Prior to her admission the fever had been attributed to her neoplasia.

Upon dental examination, extensive caries was noted in the maxillary left second bicuspid. The following tests were performed:

Tooth: Maxillary	*Tests*		
Left	*Percussion*	*Electric pulp*	*Cold*
Canine	*Normal*	*3.0*	*No Response*
First bicuspid	*Normal*	*2.0*	*No Response*
Second bicuspid	++	*2.0*	++

Based upon these tests, a diagnosis of irreversible pulpitis in the maxillary left second bicuspid was made. No radiographic evidence of periapical pathology was noted. A pulpectomy was performed the same day; completion of the endodontics was postponed. The patient's fever subsided the next day, and she was asymptomatic in this region. Induction therapy was begun that day; the hospital course was noncomplicated. Complete remission was achieved 29 days later; the endodontic procedure was completed at this time.

This case demonstrates the clinical situation in which the cancer patient presents with signs and symptoms of irreversible pulpitis but also must receive myelosuppressive chemotherapy as soon as possible. The concern is how best to manage the patient's oral complaint and concurrently minimize risk of complications secondary to that management. Recently developed guidelines have proven useful in resolving dilemmas such as this and are summarized below [54].

If there is no radiographic evidence of periapical disease, but symptoms of irreversible pulpitis are present, endodontic therapy initiated and completed during one appointment is associated with a favorable dental prognosis. However, if one cannot complete the procedure at one visit, initial biomechanical preparation and use of bacteriostatic agents often results in patient relief and does not appear to predispose the patient to acute infectious complications during subsequent myelosuppression. In this latter case, the endodontic therapy can be completed after the patient has attained complete remission. However, if the patient is symptomatic with periapical pathology and is about to undergo myelosuppression, no clear guidelines exist determining whether endodontic therapy or extraction is most beneficial. If possible, scheduled chemotherapy might be delayed to permit treatment of the acute dental infection.

The less critical case concerns the cancer patient who presents for chemotherapy with asymptomatic pulpal disease with or without asymptomatic periapical pathology. In this case, unless all endodontic care can be completed by one week prior to granulocytes becoming <1,000/μl, it appears that delaying all endodontic treatment until remission will not place the patient at substantial risk for acute sequelae.

These guidelines, then, are based chiefly upon patient symptoms; we have found that such findings, although subjective, usually supply sufficient evidence upon which to base clinical decisions.

DENTAL EXTRACTIONS

As previously noted, some clinicians have advocated full-mouth extractions for leukemic patients in remission [31]; such a radical approach is not generally accepted. However, selected extraction of teeth under appropriate circumstances is an effective means by which potential infection sites in the oral cavity can be eliminated.

Although our study found that even in a patient with severe periodontal disease pre-chemotherapy dental scaling and polishing can be an effective means by which acute periodontal infection can be prevented, teeth grossly involved with caries and/or periodontal disease should be extracted at some point. If the following guidelines are used, it appears such teeth can be safely extracted prior to onset of myelosuppression (table 5–3) [55]:

1. antibiotic prophylaxis if the patient's granulocyte count is <2,000/μl.
2. use of matched-platelet transfusions if platelet count is <40,000/μl.
3. consideration of limitations of intraalveolar hemostatic packing agents.
4. primary closure and alveolectomy at time of surgery.
5. if possible, waiting at least ten days between extraction date and induction of granulocytopenia (<1,000/μl) secondary to chemotherapy.

Most critical is the time interval between the extraction and onset of granulocytopenia. If 10 days are not possible and the patient is acutely symptomatic, one might consider delay of chemotherapy as long as possible. The importance of this delay is that, once primary epithelialization of the extraction wound occurs, the portal of entry of exogenous organisms is markedly reduced. In our experience, leaving such a wound open during periods of profound myelosuppression can lead to serious infectious complications, which, when established in the tooth socket, can be extremely difficult to manage.

Table 5–3. Oral surgical procedures in patients with ANLL

	Patient status	
	Complete remission	Admitted for treatment
Number of patients	8	20
Extractions	40	79
Surgical	2	11
Alveolectomies	9	8
Complications	1	0

SUMMARY

It is clear that complications arising from the dentition and its supporting structures can frequently arise in the myelosuppressed cancer patient. Therefore every patient about to undergo cancer chemotherapy resulting in such suppression should receive a thorough oral evaluation. In addition, the oral cavity should be considered a possible site of origin for systemic infection in these patients, even when the acute localized oral signs of inflammation are minimal. Further controlled clinical and laboratory investigations are necessary to broaden our understanding of these oral complications, including their prevention, recognition, and management.

REFERENCES

1. Schimpff SC, Young VM, Greene WH, Vermeulen GD, Moody MR, Wiernik PH: Origin of infection in acute nonlymphocytic leukemia: significance of hospital acquisition of potential pathogens. Ann Intern Med 77:707–714, 1972.
2. Levine AS, Schimpff SC, Graw RG, Young RC: Hematologic malignancies and other marrow failure states: progress in the management of complicating infections. Semin Hematol 11:141–202, 1974.
3. Gillespie GM: Renewal of buccal epithelium. Oral Surg 27:83–89, 1969.
4. Bottomley WK, Perlin E, Ross GR: Antineoplastic agents and their oral manifestations. Oral Surg 44:-527–534, 1977.
5. Dreizen S: Stomatotoxic manifestations of cancer chemotherapy. J Prosthet Dent 40:650–655, 1978.
6. Lindquist SF, Hickey AJ, Drane JB: Effect of oral hygiene on stomatitis in patients receiving cancer chemotherapy. J Prosthet Dent 40:312–314, 1978.
7. Beck S: Impact of a systematic oral care protocol on stomatitis after chemotherapy. Cancer Nurs 2:185–199, 1979.
8. Dreizen S, McCredie KB, Dicke KA, Zander AR, Peters LJ: Oral complications of bone marrow transplantation in adults with acute leukemia. Postgrad Med 66:187–196, 1979.
9. Daeffler R: Oral hygiene measures for patients with cancer (I). Cancer Nurs 3:347–356, 1980.
10. Ostchega Y: Preventing and treating cancer chemotherapy's oral complications. Nursing 10:47–52, 1980.
11. Daeffler R: Oral hygiene measures for patients with cancer (II). Cancer Nurs 3:427–432, 1980.
12. Daeffler R: Oral hygiene measures for patients with cancer (III). Cancer Nurs 4:29–35, 1981.
13. Dreizen S: Chemotherapy-induced oral mucositis in adult leukemia. Postgrad Med 69:103–112, 1981.
14. Hickey AJ, Toth BB, Lindquist SB: Effect of intravenous hyperalimentation and oral care on the development of oral stomatitis during cancer chemotherapy. J Prosthet Dent 47:188–193, 1982.
15. Loesche WJ: Bacterial succession in dental plaque: role in dental disease. In *Microbiology—1975,* Schlessinger D (ed), Washington, D.C., American Society of Microbiologists, 1975:132–136.
16. Page RC, Schroeder HE: Pathogenesis of inflammatory periodontal disease. Lab Invest 34:235–249, 1976.
17. Goldman HM, Cohn DW: *Periodontal Therapy,* 4th ed., St. Louis, C.V. Mosby Co, 1968, p. 64.
18. Segelman AE, Doku HC: Treatment of the oral complications of leukemia. J Oral Surg 35:469–477, 1977.
19. Sonis ST, Sonis AL, Lieberman A: Oral complications in patients receiving treatment for malignancies other than of the head and neck. J Am Dent Assoc 97:468–472, 1978.
20. Lockhart PB, Sonis ST: Relationship of oral complications to peripheral blood leukocyte and platelet counts in patients receiving cancer chemotherapy. Oral Surg 48:21–28, 1979.
21. Peterson DE, Overholser CD: Dental management of leukemic patients. Oral Surg 47:40–42, 1979.
22. Sonis A, Sonis S: Oral complications of cancer chemotherapy in pediatric patients. J Periodontal 3:122–128, 1979.
23. Peterson DE, Overholser CD: Increased morbidity associated with oral infection in patients with acute nonlymphocytic leukemia. Oral Surg 51:390–393, 1981.
24. Greenberg MS, Cohen SG, McKitrick JC, Cassileth PA: The oral flora as a source of septicemia in patients with acute leukemia. Oral Surg 53:32–36, 1982.
25. Overholser CD, Peterson DE, Williams LT, Schimpff SC: Periodontal infection in patients with acute nonlymphocytic leukemia: prevalence of acute exacerbations. Arch Intern Med 142:551–554, 1982.
26. Johanson WG, Pierce AK, Sanford JP: Changing pharyngeal bacterial flora of hospitalized patients. N Engl J Med 281:1137–1140, 1969.
27. Brown LR, Mackler BF, Levy BM, et al.: Comparison of the plaque microflora in immunodeficient and immunocompetent dental patients. J Dent Res 58:2344–2352, 1979.

28. Brown LR, Dreizen S, Bodey GP: Effect of immunosuppression on the human oral flora. In *Comparative Immunology of the Oral Cavity,* Mergenhagen SE, Scherp HW (eds), Washington, D.C., U.S. Government Printing Office, 1973, pp. 204–220.
29. Schimpff SC, Aisner J, Wiernik PH: Infection in acute nonlymphocytic leukemia: the alimentary canal as a major source of pathogens. In *New Criteria for Antimicrobial Therapy: Maintenance of Digestive Tract Colonization Resistance,* van der Waaij D, Verhoef J (eds), Amsterdam, Excerpta Medica, 1979, pp 12–29.
30. Newman KA, Schimpff SC, Young VM, Wiernik PH: Lessons learned from surveillance cultures in patients with acute nonlymphocytic leukemia. Am J Med 70:423–431, 1981.
31. Chapman RM, Crosby WH: Elective dental extraction in leukemia (letter). N Engl J Med 295:114, 1976.
32. Parfitt GJ: Cleansing the subgingival space. J Periodontol 34:133–139, 1963.
33. Vollmer DE: Preventive dentistry: precaution pays. J Am Soc Prev Dent 4:31–33, 1974.
34. Schimpff SC, Satterlee W, Young VM, Serpick A: Empiric therapy with carbenicillin and gentamicin for febrile patients with cancer and granulocytopenia. N Engl J Med 284:1061–1065, 1971.
35. Bodey GP, Buckley M, Sathe YS, Freireich EJ: Quantitative relationships between circulating leukocytes and infection in patients with acute leukemia. Ann Intern Med 64:328–340, 1966.
36. Sickles EA, Greene WH, Wiernik PH: Clinical presentation of infection in granulocytopenic patients. Arch Intern Med 135:715–719, 1975.
37. Greene JC, Vermillion JR: The simplified oral hygiene index. J Am Dent Assoc 68:7–13, 1964.
38. Schimpff SC: Therapy of infection in patients with granulocytopenia. Med Clin North Am 1101–1118, 1977.
39. Cobe HM: Transitory bacteremia. Oral Surg 7:609–615, 1954.
40. Conner HD, Haberman S, Collings CK, Winford TE: Bacteremias following periodontal scaling in patients with healthy appearing gingiva. J Periodontal 38:22–28, 1967.
41. Lineberger LT, DeMarco TJ: Evaluation of transient bacteremia following routine periodontal procedures. J Periodontol 44:757–762, 1973.
42. Sconyers JR, Crawford JJ, Moriarity JD: Relationship of bacteremia to toothbrushing in patients with periodontitis. J Am Dent Assoc 87:616–622, 1973.
43. Wank HA, Levinson ME, Rose LF, Cohen DW: A quantitative measurement of bacteremia and its relationship to plaque control. J Periodontol 47:683–686, 1976.
44. Silver JG, Martin AW, McBride BC: Experimental transient bacteraemias in human subjects with varying degrees of plaque accumulation and gingival inflammation. J Clin Periodontol 4:92–99, 1977.
45. Silver JC, Martin AW, McBride BC: Experimental transient bacteraemias in human subjects with clinically healthy gingivae. J Clin Periodontol 6:33–36, 1979.
46. Carroll GC, Sebor RJ: Dental flossing and its relationship to transient bacteremia. J Periodontol 51:691–692, 1980.
47. Berger SA, Weitzman S, Edberg SC, Casey JI: Bacteremia after the use of an oral irrigation device. Ann Intern Med 80:510–511, 1974.
48. Kremer WB, Vogler WR, Chan YK: An attempt at synchronization of marrow cells in acute leukemia. Cancer 37:390–403, 1976.
49. Kansal V, Omura GA, Soong SJ: Prognosis in adult acute myelogenous leukemia related to performance status and other factors. Cancer 38:329–334, 1976.
50. Peterson DE, Overholser CD, Williams LT, Newman KA, Schimpff SC, Wiernik PH. Acute periodontal infection at admission in acute nonlymphocytic leukemia patients. Proc Am Fed Clin Res 30:422A, 1982.
51. Suzuki JB, DePaola LG, Nauman RK: Periodontal therapy in a patient on cancer chemotherapy. J Am Dent Assoc 104:473–475, 1982.
52. Weekly Clinicopathological Exercises, Case 36-1977. N Engl J Med 297:546–551, 1977.
53. Levinson SL, Barondess JA: Occult dental infection as a cause of fever of obscure origin. Am J Med 66:463–467, 1979.
54. Peterson DE, Overholser CD, Williams LT: Endodontic therapy in patients receiving myelosuppressive chemotherapy. Proc J Dent Res 61:276, 1982.
55. Overholser CD, Peterson DE, Bergman SA: Dental extractions in patients with leukemia. J Oral Surg 40:296–298, 1982.

6. ORAL COMPLICATIONS OF BONE-MARROW TRANSPLANTATION

MARK M. SCHUBERT, D.D.S., M.S.D.
KEITH M. SULLIVAN, M.D.
KENNETH T. IZUTSU, PhD.
EDMOND L. TRUELOVE, D.D.S., M.S.D.

OVERVIEW

Introduction

The techniques for bone-marrow transplantation grew out of the studies by Jacobson, et al. [1] and Lorenz et al. [2], first reported in 1950. They showed that lethally irradiated mice could survive if the spleen was adequately shielded or if an infusion of bone-marrow cells was given. Initial efforts in man to utilize the technique of marrow infusion following lethal radiation demonstrated the potential usefulness of this technique but were generally unsuccessful. In the late 1950s two leukemia patients given supralethal radiation demonstrated successful engraftment after marrow infusion from identical twin donors but later succumbed to recurrent disease [3]. With the advances in kidney transplantation in the 1960s, the role of histocompatability matching between donor and recipient was appreciated. Elucidation of the histocompatability leukocyte antigen (HLA) complex facilitated marrow transplantation between HLA-identical siblings. In the early 1970s marrow transplantation was further enhanced with the development of better supportive care for patients following marrow ablation.

Today the survival rates for marrow recipients are steadily improving and the use of transplantation as a therapeutic means of treating acute leukemia, aplastic anemia, and severe combined immunodeficiency is meeting with increasing success. Severe aplastic anemia

This work was supported in part by Grant numbers CA 18029, CA 30924, CA 18221, and CA 15704 awarded by the National Cancer Institute, DHHS. Dr. Sullivan was supported in part by a Junior Faculty Clinical Fellowship from the American Cancer Society. Dr. Izutsu is supported by NIH Grant DE 02600.

D.E. Peterson and S.T. Sonis (eds.), ORAL COMPLICATIONS OF CANCER CHEMOTHERAPY, 93-112.

(marrow failure) has a mortality of 50% within six months of diagnosis and less than 20% are alive after one year in spite of conventional transfusion and antibiotic supportive care. An international study found marrow transplant to be the treatment of choice in severe aplastic anemia [4]. Since 1976 the Seattle transplant team has reported 70–80% five-year survival in patients receiving HLA-matched allogeneic marrow grafts [5,6]. The results in patients with acute leukemia are also improving steadily, with as many as 55% of patients with acute nonlymphoblastic leukemia in first remission surviving free of leukemia five years after allogeneic transplantation [7]. In addition, marrow transplantation has been shown to successfully eradicate the malignant clone of Philadelphia chromosome positive cells in patients with chronic granulocytic leukemia and results in long-term disease-free survivors [8].

Candidates for marrow transplantation have disorders that either involve the marrow such that survival depends on establishing a new marrow or require such aggressive treatment that a normal marrow would be irreversibly damaged, thereby limiting therapy. Marrow from the donor provides myeloid, lymphoid, and macrophage stem cells to reestablish the defective or damaged marrow. For obvious ethical reasons the clinical practice of marrow transplantation began with seriously ill patients with refractory, end-stage diseases. While early studies selected identical-twin donors, the majority of transplants over the last ten years have been from HLA identical siblings. More recently, selected HLA mismatched donors (family members with only one identical genetic haplotype) or even phenotypically identical but unrelated donors have been utilized as advances in the understanding of transplantation biology and immunogenetics have been realized [9]. Bone-marrow transplantation has become more than just an experimental procedure and may be considered a reasonable primary or alternative treatment for a variety of otherwise-lethal disorders [10].

Principles of marrow transplantation

Donor selection

The three types of marrow donors are defined by their genetic similarity to the recipient.

Autologous marrow grafting involves removing a patient's own bone marrow, cryopreserving it during intensive (otherwise lethal) myelosuppresive chemoradiotherapy, and then returning the stored marrow to the patient to allow reestablishment of a functioning marrow. Tumors considered for treatment by this technique must be sensitive to the high dose of chemotherapy and radiation and it is hoped not involve the bone marrow. Such disorders include Hodgkin's disease and non-Hodgkin's lymphomas, small-cell lung cancers, and testicular and ovarian carcinomas.

Syngeneic marrow from a monozygous (identical) twin offers a source of marrow free of differences of transplantation antigens that may mediate complications such as graft-versus-host disease. In addition, some twins have been cured of aplastic anemia with simple marrow infusion from their twin without immunosuppressive preparative chemotherapy before transplant [11].

Allogeneic marrow transplantation employs a family member donor (usually sibling) who shares all or carefully selected portions of the HLA complex [12]. The genetic loci that make up the HLA region are located on chromosome 6 and encode an array of antigens known as a haplotype. Each parent provides one haplotype to each offspring and the chances are about one in four that siblings will be HLA-identical. HLA-A, -B, and -C are detected by serological techniques utilizing a microcytotoxicity assay. A mixed leukocyte culture (MLC) is used to detect HLA-D. Several other genetic loci related to HLA-D have been recognized to contribute to the HLA region and these are serologically detected by typing B-lymphocytes. Advances in tissue typing will undoubtedly detect other HLA loci of importance in transplant matching.

Pretransplant conditioning

The aims of preparative conditioning of the marrow recipient with chemotherapy and total body irradiation are to eliminate malignant cells and/or prevent graft rejection. Allogeneic marrow transplant recipients, except for infants with severe combined immunologic deficiency, are immunologically capable of rejecting a marrow graft that is not identical to their own. Consequently, agents are used prior to grafting that will suppress this immune reaction. The most common regimens are discussed below [13].

APLASTIC ANEMIA. Patients usually receive large doses (200 mg/kg) of cyclophosphamide, a potent chemotherapeutic agent with significant immunosuppressive properties. Many transplant centers also employ varying doses of total body irradiation in the preparation.

ACUTE LEUKEMIA. Pretransplant conditioning for leukemia patients requires that all malignant cells be destroyed. To achieve this, most transplant centers use a high-dose chemoradiotherapy regimen. For example, the Seattle group uses Cyclophosphamide (120 mg/kg) plus single dose (1,000 rad) or fractionated (1,200–1,575 rad) total body irradiation. Radiation doses of this magnitude are approximately two-and-one-half times the lethal dose (LD_{100}) for marrow ablation. Besides eradicating malignant cells, this regimen will also provide the needed immunosuppression.

Bone-marrow infusion and engraftment

Marrow is obtained from the donor under general or spinal anesthesia by multiple aspirations from the pelvic bones. A volume of 500 to 800 ml is obtained and mixed with a heparinized solution of tissue culture medium. The collected marrow is passed through fine screens to break up marrow aggregates. On the average between $2\text{–}6 \times 10^8$ marrow cells per kg of patient weight are administered via an intravenous infusion [14]. The donor stem-cell graft migrates to the marrow spaces of the host and proliferates to establish a functional marrow.

The marrow is infused after completion of chemoradiotherapy preparation of the recipient; the day of the transplant is designated day 0. Following the transplant preparation, circulating white blood cells (WBCs), granulocytes, red blood cells (RBCs), and platelets rapidly fall with WBC and granulocyte counts approaching zero. It is necessary to support patients during this period with platelet and RBC transfusions. Patients are extremely susceptible to infections and bleeding following marrow ablation. Acute toxicity of the preparative regimen begins to resolve, and between days 20 and 30 evidence of engraftment is detected by increased peripheral WBC and platelet counts. Engraftment is substantiated by return of cellularity on marrow aspirations, and cytogenetic and/or red cell genetic

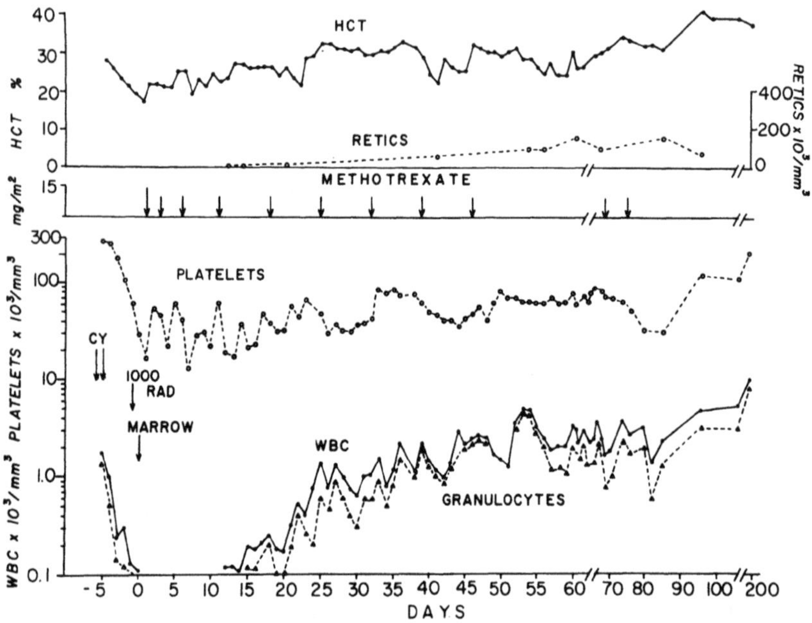

Figure 6–1. Hematological events in a leukemia patient treated with bone-marrow transplantation. Pretransplant conditioning consisted of two doses of cyclophosphamide (Cy), 60 mg/Kg each, and 1,000 rads of total-body-irradiation. Marrow from an HLA-identical sibling was infused on Day 0. Platelet transfusions were given between days 6 and 27. The ordinate is on a log scale. Changes in hematocrit (HCT), reticulocytes (retics), platelets, white blood cells (WBC), and granulocytes are shown.

markers confirm that the regenerating marrow is of donor origin. Figure 6–1 shows the hematologic events following marrow transplantation.

Supportive care of patients following transplant

Until a patient's graft is fully functional it is critical to provide extensive supportive care. Besides improved management of preexisting infections, more effective techniques for preventing endogenous and exogenous infections have been developed in recent years [15]. Patients may be placed in protective isolation. Studies have shown complete isolation in a laminar-air-flow room with skin sterilization, sterile diet, and gut decontamination with nonabsorbable oral antibiotics to be effective in preventing bacterial infection [16]. In addition, granulocyte transfusions to maintain a granulocyte count above $200/mm^3$ may also be used and have been advocated for both prophylactic and therapeutic purposes [17].

Infectious complications are a major problem following transplant [15]. During the first 30 days posttransplant when granulocyte counts are lowest, bacterial or fungal infections can be a significant problem. With the profound loss of granulocytes during this period, the classic signs of the inflammatory process are often absent and fever is most often the primary indicator of infection. Once granulocytes begin to recover around day 30, viral infections may predominate. Infections due to herpes simplex virus, varicella zoster virus, and cytomegalovirus are frequently noted. Upwards of 50% of all marrow transplant patients develop varicella zoster virus infections and the median time of onset is five months posttransplantation. Bacterial and fungal infections do overlap in this period, especially in instances where granulocyte counts are slow to recover. After day 100 the frequency of infections dramatically decreases; the major exception is in patients with chronic graft-vs-host disease who continue to have profound immune deficiencies.

Systemic antibiotics are required when patients with severe neutropenia become febrile and are maintained until an unsupported granulocyte count of over $500/mm^3$ is achieved. If fever persists and no bacterial organisms are isolated, antifungal therapy may be initiated. Acyclovir, an effective antiviral agent, has been recently found to be useful in controlling some types of viral infections in marrow graft recipients [18].

Platelet and RBC transfusions are administered until the graft is self-supporting, and fluid and electrolyte balance is carefully monitored following transplantation. The conditioning regimen invariably causes nausea, vomiting, and oral mucositis which can severely limit oral intake for several weeks. To provide nutritional support and central venous access, a Hickman catheter is inserted before starting chemotherapy [19]. Through this line hyperalimentation as well as blood products and intravenous medications can be given.

Graft rejection

Graft rejection may be encountered in patients with aplastic anemia [20]. It is believed that this immunologic process results from sensitization to previous blood transfusions. Accordingly, studies of untransfused patients with aplastic anemia have shown a significantly lower rejection rate. More intense pretransplant immunosuppressive conditioning or posttransplant unirradiated donor buffy coat transfusions have reduced rejection rates [4].

Leukemic relapse

The problem of malignant recurrence is one central to the treatment of any malignant disease and prevention depends on eradication of all malignant cells. This problem is especially true for patients with leukemia in relapse at the time of transplant [21]. One approach has been to increase the dose of total body irradiation by fractionation of the irradiation. Relapses following allogeneic transplantation are infrequent when patients with acute nonlymphoblastic leukemia are transplanted in first remission [7]. This may be due to decreased numbers of residual leukemia cells, the presence of leukemic cells not yet resistant to therapeutic agents, or both.

Graft-versus-host disease

Graft-versus-host disease is an immunologic reaction mounted by engrafted lymphoid cells (probably T-cells) against transplantation antigens of host tissues. Two forms of graft-versus-host disease have been identified. One is an acute form that occurs in the first several months posttransplant and usually involves the skin, gastrointestinal tract, and/or liver [21,22]. The second form is known as chronic graft-versus-host disease and can develop as an extension of acute graft-versus-host disease or de novo several months after transplant [23]. The manifestations of chronic graft-versus-host disease include skin disease, keratoconjunctivitis, oral mucositis, esophageal or vaginal strictures, intestinal involvement, pulmonary insufficiency, chronic liver disease, and generalized wasting. It has been noted to resemble a variety of naturally occurring systemic collagen vascular diseases such as scleroderma, lupus erythematosus, lichen planus, and Sjögren's syndrome. Both forms of graft-versus-host disease can cause severe immunologic deficiency and result in fatal infections [24].

Efforts to prevent graft-versus-host disease have centered around immunosuppressive therapy. Methotrexate has been used routinely after the transplant in an attempt to prevent or ameliorate graft-versus-host disease [11]. Methotrexate is given intravenously at a dose of 15 mg/m^2 on day 1 posttransplant and 10 mg/m^2 on days 3, 6, 11, 18, and then weekly through day 102. More recently cyclosporin A (a fungal metabolite with potent immunosuppressive properties) has shown encouraging results in preventing or delaying graft-versus-host disease [25].

Treatment of established acute graft-versus-host disease has met with varying success. Despite prophylactic methotrexate, approximately 35% of allogeneic marrow transplant patients will develop moderate to severe (Grade II–IV) acute graft-versus-host disease and between one-fourth and one-third of these patients die of graft-versus-host disease-related complications [26]. Antithymocyte globulin and/or prednisone have been used with some success.

Chronic graft-versus-host disease develops in 25 to 40% of long-term survivors of allogeneic transplantation [27]. Recently the Seattle team has reported the use of combination immunosuppressive therapy to treat chronic graft-versus-host disease. Using prednisone in combination with procarbazine, cyclophosphamide, or azathioprine, 71% of the chronic graft-versus-host disease patients treated had long-term disability-free survival [27]. Despite these encouraging results, however, more effective regimens to prevent or treat graft-versus-host disease need to be sought.

Immunologic recovery and tolerance

During the first three to nine months following marrow transplantation, patients have little or no natural means to fight opportunistic infections. Efforts to prevent or treat graft-versus-host disease further compromise immunologic function. Studies of immune function have shown similar patterns of recovery in both syngeneic and allogeneic recipients. The total lymphocyte (T and B cell), granulocyte, and platelet counts approach normal by the end of the first month but other immunologic parameters remain profoundly impaired [28]. At one year postgrafting patients without graft-versus-host disease have recovered near-normal immune function and are free of infections. Chronic graft-versus-host disease patients, however, may exhibit severe immunodeficiency for as long as the graft-versus-host disease remains active [29]. Prophylactic antibiotic therapy with trimethoprim-sulfamethoxazole is given to patients with active chronic graft-versus-host disease [27].

A long-term healthy survivor of bone-marrow transplantation has myeloid, lymphocyte, and monocyte-macrophage cells of donor origin. These cells of graft origin are tolerant of the host tissues and a variety of theories have been developed to explain this phenomena. Some of the mechanisms proposed involve central tolerance, tolerance maintained by blocking factors, and suppressor cell induced tolerance. The elucidation of the immunologic mechanism(s) of the tolerant state will not only be of significance for marrow transplantation but possibly for our understanding of naturally occurring autoimmune disease [30,31].

ORAL COMPLICATIONS OF MARROW TRANSPLANTATION

Etiology of oral complications following marrow transplantation

The oral cavity is a frequent site of complications during bone-marrow transplantation. The severity of problems ranges from transient discomfort from oral mucositis to potentially life-threatening situations from fulminant infections. The oral-tissue damage encountered during marrow grafting often results from the additive effects of several different insults, and it is this combination of effects that makes the marrow transplant patient unique.

The chemoradiotherapy conditioning regimens are the foremost contributors to oral breakdown [32–35]. For example, cyclophosphamide is an alkylating agent known to cause mucosal atrophy and ulceration as well as interfere with collagen formation and granulocyte bacterial killing [36]. Methotrexate, a folic acid antagonist, causes thinning and ulceration of mucosal epithelium and collagen degradation [37]. The effects of ionizing irradiation on oral tissues are known to include generalized mucosal atrophy, ulceration, vasculitis, salivary gland inflammation, and damage leading to xerostomia [34].

When these agents are used in combination during the marrow grafting procedure it is clear why the oral cavity is at such high risk for breakdown. With the loss of the protective barrier function of the oral epithelium, development of granulocytopenia, and loss of protection provided by saliva and its constituent products (mucins, IgA, lactoferrin, lactoperoxidase) the oral tissues are susceptible to a variety of fungal, viral, and bacterial infections. The use of high-dose broad-spectrum antibiotics further modifies the oral flora and allows pathogenic as well as opportunistic organisms to flourish [15,38,39]. The nutritional status of the patient can be altered by drugs or graft-versus-host disease, further interfering with normal mucosal proliferation and healing. The result is an organ whose functional integrity has been severely compromised such that normal physical, chemical, and infectious challenges are poorly tolerated.

Manifestations of oral disorders

The type, timing, and severity of oral involvement can vary significantly from patient to patient. When considering oral management strategies, it is convenient to divide marrow transplantation therapy into four phases. Phase I starts at the time of hospital admission and includes pretransplant workup and chemoradiotherapy preparation. Phase II begins at the time of marrow infusion (day 0) and extends up to the time that engraftment has occurred and granulocytes reappear. Patients are discharged from the hospital with adequate granulocyte counts around day 30–35. Phase III includes outpatient follow-up over the next 60 days at the transplant center. Phase IV covers the period of long-term follow-up examinations after the patient has regained immunologic function.

Phase I

Oral complications encountered during this period represent dental problems acquired prior to transplantation. Patients may have extensive dental breakdown with chronic abscesses, root tips, and so on, having avoided dental care because of their previous medical problems. Fortunately, physicians are becoming more aware of the role of proper dental care in the management of the patient with hematologic disorders.

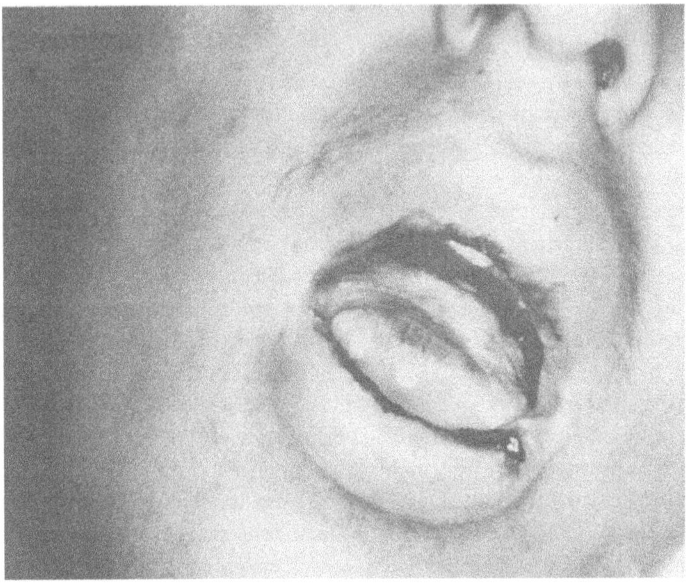

Figure 6–2. Phase II: Severe mucositis in a bone-marrow-transplant patient (day 10).

Phase II

Between four and ten days elapse before the full effects of chemotherapy are clinically manifest. Oral breakdown from these agents is not evident until after day 0. Severe symptoms may persist until day 20–30 when engraftment and resolution of neutropenia is achieved. Patients receiving total body irradiation in the preparative regimen transiently develop bilateral parotitis and may develop more significant mucositis and xerostomia than patients receiving only cyclophosphamide. Mucositis, ulceration, hemorrhage, infection, and xerostomia are common [40] (figure 6–2). The mucosal abnormalities will initially appear as atrophy with generalized erythema noted in the nonkeratinized surfaces of the buccal and labial mucosa, floor of mouth, ventral tongue, and soft palate. As these effects become more apparent the para- and ortho-keratinized mucosal surfaces also will become atrophic. Ulcerations will appear as either discrete shallow lesions, or may represent large eroded areas which often become secondarily infected or covered by a thick greyish-yellow pseudomembrane. The most common sites for ulcerations are the lateral borders of the tongue, floor of the mouth/ventral tongue, and buccal mucosa, but all mucosal surfaces can be involved (figure 6–3).

Most oral infections during this period are bacterial or fungal in origin. Inflammatory reactions are not profound due to the severe neutropenia. Oral bacterial infections are often non-descript and an accurate diagnosis depends on the results of cultures. Oral candida infections are common and are usually of the acute pseudomembranous type. Herpetic (herpes simplex virus and varicella zoster virus) infections can present with crops of vesicles

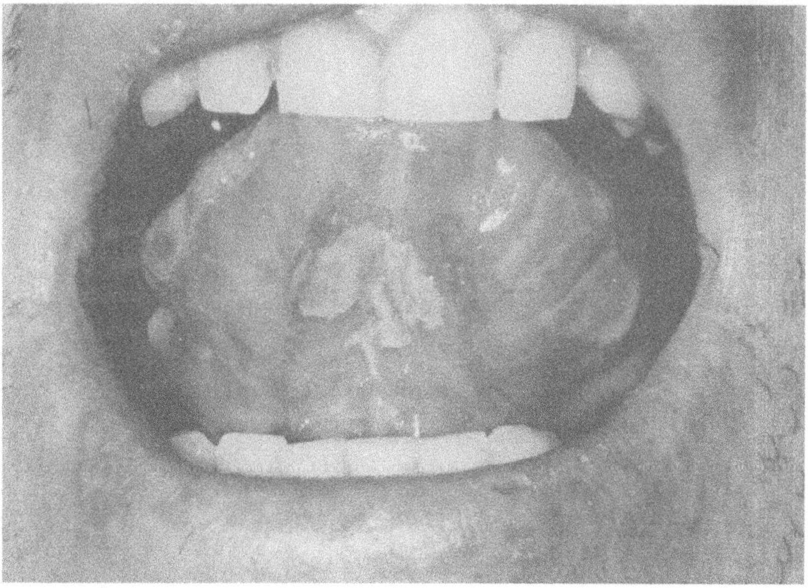

Figure 6–3. Phase II: Ulcerative mucositis on ventral and lateral surface of the tongue on day 7 posttransplant for a 34-year-old acute leukemia patient.

which rapidly rupture leaving small ulcers that may coalesce. Often it is difficult to differentiate mucosal breakdown due to conditioning agents from viral infection (figure 6–4). Involvement of perioral tissues (lips and nose) with lesions helps in clinical assessments, but diagnosis depends ultimately on the results of viral cultures. Studies have shown that the more severe mucositis is, the more likely it is that the patient is excreting herpes simplex virus [15]. These viral-induced lesions are slow-healing and improvement may not be seen until granulocyte counts increase (figure 6–5). Methotrexate can also amplify oral breakdown. When cyclosporin A is used instead of methotrexate to prevent graft-versus-host disease, severity and extent of mucositis appears lessened. Gingival hypertrophy has not been observed as it has in renal transplant patients receiving the drug [41].

Phase III

Gradual oral improvement is noted during this phase, though the rate of recovery can be highly variable. As early as day 50–60 posttransplant, some patients will have complete healing of oral lesions. In others, xerostomia will persist in varying degrees for as long as six to eight months posttransplant. Persistent oral problems are especially common among the 25–40% of long-term survivors who develop chronic graft-versus-host disease [27,42]. Approximately 80% of patients with the extensive form of chronic graft-versus-host disease will develop oral involvement [27]. Subjective complaints in chronic graft-versus-host disease patients include xerostomia and stomatitis. A clue to oral involvement with chronic graft-versus-host disease is the presence of increasing xerostomia and/or generalized

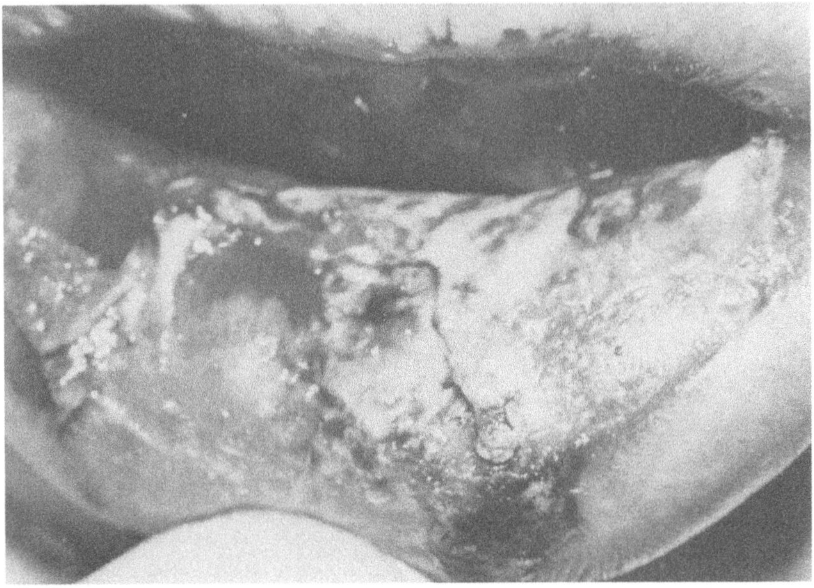

Figure 6–4. Phase II: Hemorrhagic and ulcerative mucositis in a bone-marrow transplant patient on day 8. The patient had culture positive herpes simplex lesions and continued to excrete virus for 10 days. These lesions took over 35 days to heal.

stomatitis around day 100. Toothpastes and acidic foods are frequently reported to cause pain and oral irritation. Clinical findings include mucosal erythema and lichen planus-like and lupus-like lesions. Lichenoid reactions can range from fine white reticular striae on otherwise normal appearing mucosa to large plaques or patches on the lateral surface of the tongue (figure 6–6). With more severe involvement erosive lichen planus-like lesions have been noted. The buccal mucosa and lateral tongue are the most commonly involved sites but lichenoid lesions have also been observed on the gingivae, hard palate, and vermillion border of the lips. Lupus-like ulcerations have been noted, with the buccal mucosa, tongue, and palate being the most commonly observed sites (figures 6–7 and 6–8). Here the ulcerations tend to be broad and have a very erythematous border and a central greyish-yellow covering. Generalized mucosal atrophy is often apparent with extensive chronic graft-versus-host disease and keratinization seems to be absent. The gingiva loses its stippling and the papilla of the tongue are lost. In addition, oral and perioral changes consistent with scleroderma have been noted (figure 6–9). Histologic studies have shown lymphocytic inflammation and necrosis involving mucosal and salivary duct epithelium [43]. The Seattle group is routinely using the results of labial mucosal and minor salivary gland biopsies to screen for and assess the course of chronic graft-versus-host disease during Phases III and IV [27,43]. A Sjögrens-like reaction has been reported in chronic graft-versus-host disease patients [44]. The extent and type of salivary gland changes occurring with chronic graft-versus-host disease are yet to be fully elucidated, but most of the salivary changes noted to date are similar to those observed in Sjögren's syndrome, that is, decreased

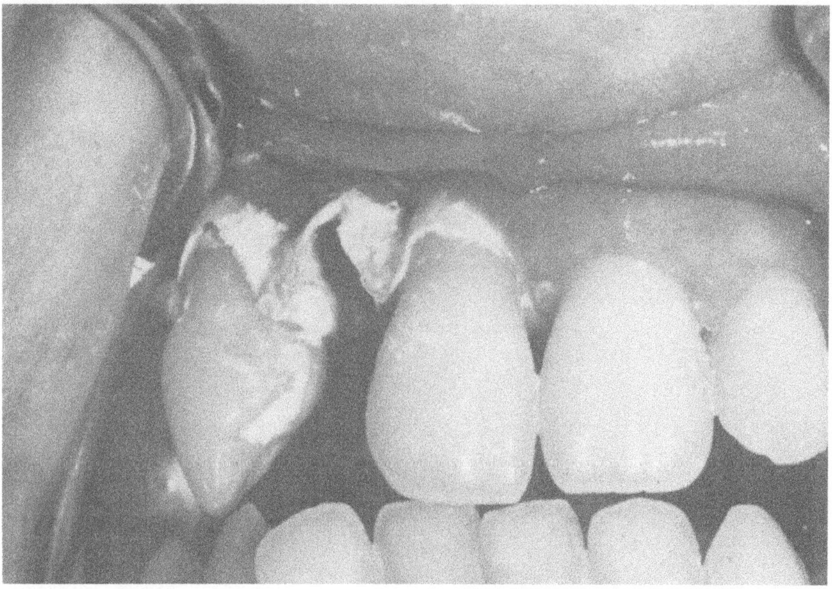

Figure 6–5. Severe herpes simplex virus involvement with secondary bacterial and fungal infection of maxillary right periodontium 25 days postmarrow transplantation. This patient ultimately lost all teeth in this quadrant.

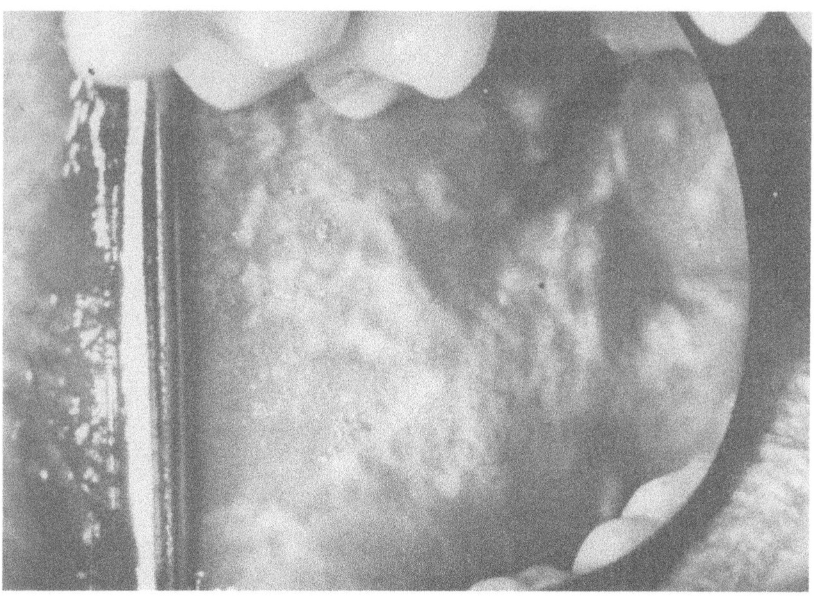

Figure 6–6. Phase III: Lichenoid lesions and striae of a patient with chronic graft-vs-host disease (day 95).

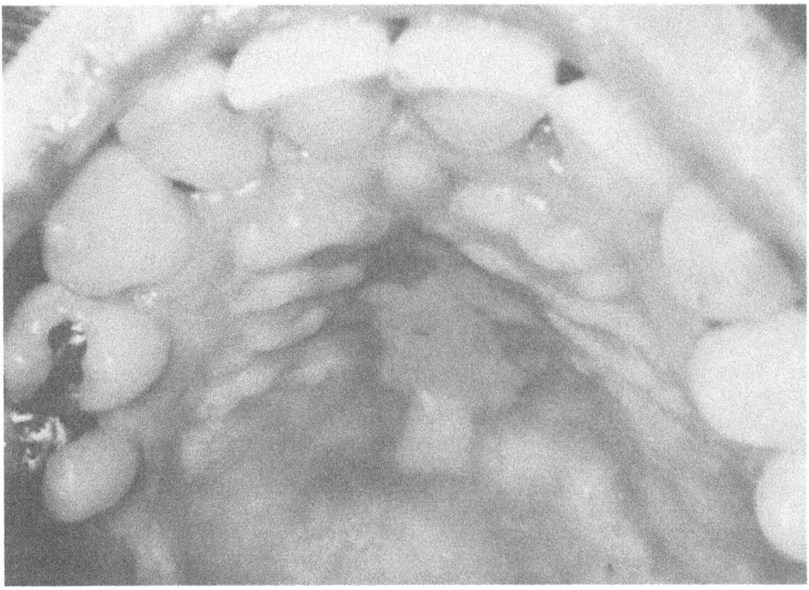

Figure 6–7. Phase IV: Lupus-like lesion on the palate of a patient with chronic graft-vs-host disease (day 375).

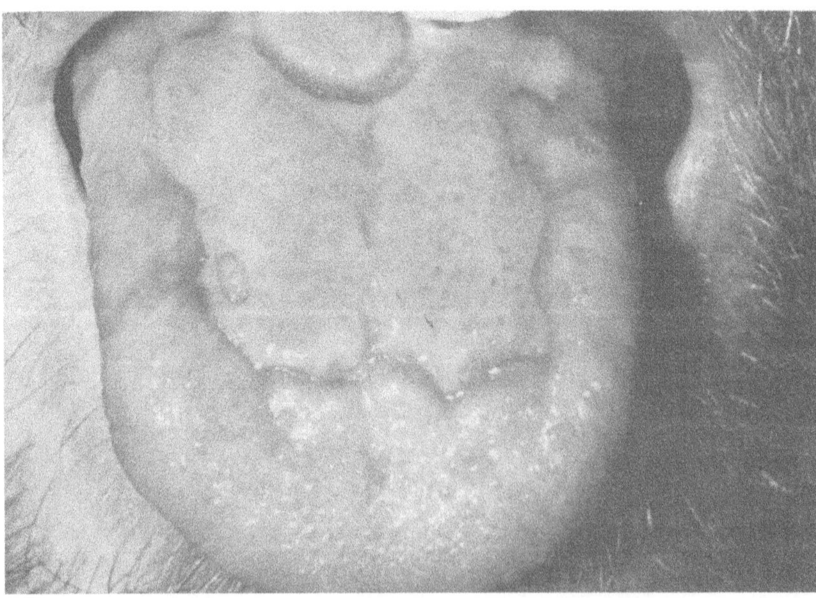

Figure 6–8. Phase IV: Lupus-like lesion on tongue of same patient in figure 6–7 (day 375).

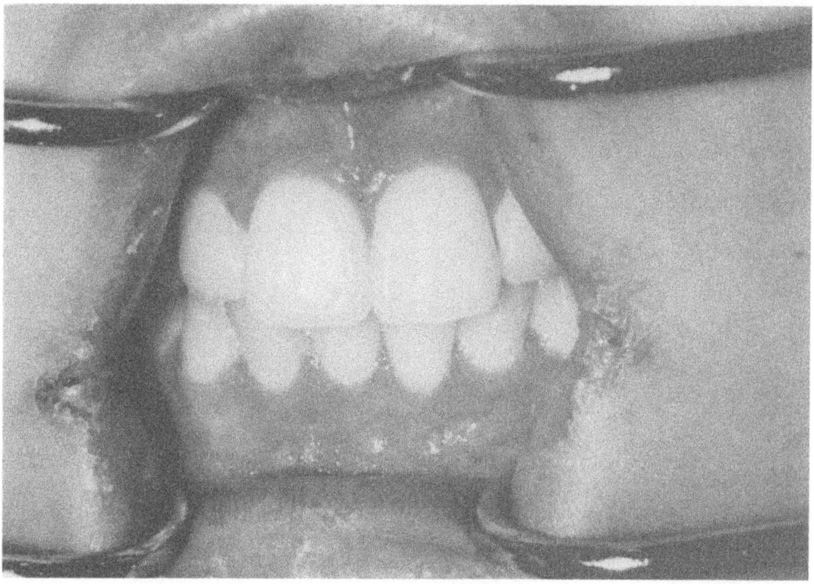

Figure 6–9. Phase IV: Patient with chronic graft-vs-host disease on day 368 with severe oral involvement. Patient had atrophic gingivae, candidial angular stomatitis, as well as skin and lip changes similar to scleroderma (that is, decreased elasticity, decreased oral opening, and temporomandibular joint fibrosis).

salivary flow rates and phosphate concentrations and elevated sodium and lysozyme concentrations [45–51]. Since similar histopathologic findings have also been made in the two conditions [43], it is likely that the salivary changes share common etiologies. Thus inflammatory processes in the gland probably cause an increased transudation of serum components into saliva, and the frequently observed sialodochitis probably results in a ductal sodium resorption defect which explains the elevation in sodium concentration [45]. The relative contributions of graft-versus-host disease and chemotherapy and total body irradiation to these inflammatory processes remain to be evaluated. However, effects due to the conditioning regimens are expected to diminsh with time following transplant.

One change that is unique to transplant recipients with chronic graft-versus-host disease is a decrease in salivary IgA levels [47]. The reported lack of intestinal IgA-bearing plasma cells of patients with acute graft-versus-host disease [52] is consistent with this salivary defect, and suggests that the mucosal immune system that is present in salivary, lacrimal, peribronchial, and intestinal secretions may be disrupted in these patients. Such a defect could account for the frequent infections observed at these sites in patients with graft-versus-host disease [24,27].

Viral infections are still common during this phase, and bacterial and fungal infections may continue to occur, especially in patients with persistent granulocytopenia (figure 6–10). Previously quiescent periapical or periodontal lesions have been noted to become active during this period of recovery. After day 100 the incidence of oral infections

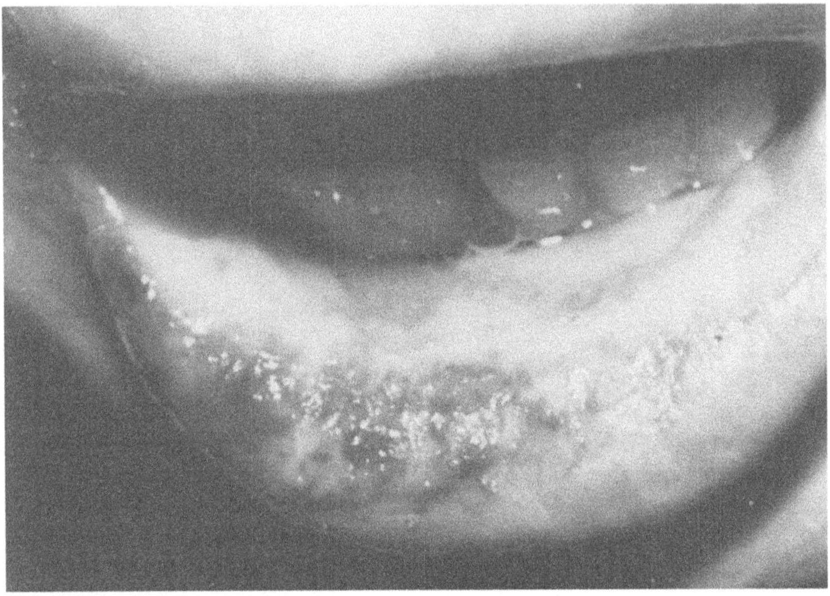

Figure 6–10. Phase III: Confluent herpes lesions with crusting on the lower lip of a patient 85 days postmarrow transplantation.

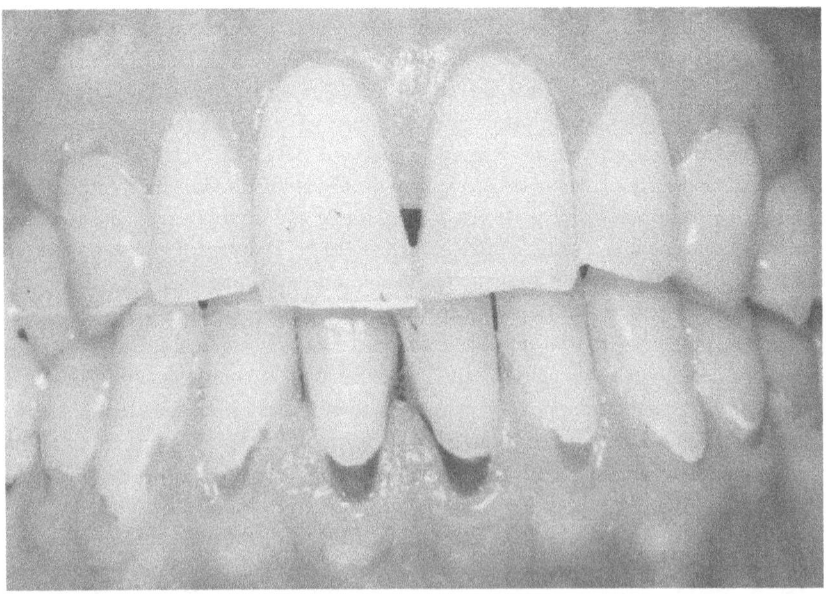

Figure 6–11. Phase IV: Rampant decay in a patient suffering severe xerostomia (day 380).

generally decreases, but this will depend on the development of chronic graft-versus-host disease.

Phase IV

The majority of long-term survivors have normal oral findings. Some will have varying degrees of xerostomia, some to the extent that rampant decay becomes a serious problem (figure 6–11). Also, it is not unusual to see delayed eruption patterns of permanent teeth in children transplanted with primary or mixed dentition, but this has not seemed to present any significant problems. Otherwise, this group of healthy survivors is unremarkable.

Patients with active chronic graft-versus-host disease being treated with immunosuppressive therapy will often be asymptomatic but continue to display objective mucosal characteristics of chronic graft-versus-host disease. Gingival tissues can be significantly affected by chronic graft-versus-host disease, and extensive periodontal breakdown has been noted where oral hygiene is inadequate. Decreased or absent salivary flow rates facilitate formation of dental caries. One ten-year-old patient with chronic graft-versus-host disease has been noted to have agenesis of root structure and cessation of eruption of permanent teeth. Whether this was due to chemotherapy, radiation, chronic graft-versus-host disease, or a combination of these factors is not clear. The problem remains an important clinical consideration for long-term dental management of children following marrow transplantation. Finally, patients with inactive extensive chronic graft-versus-host disease can present with residual atrophic changes of all oral mucosal surfaces; except for periodontal considerations, however, this does not appear to be a significant problem.

Management of oral complications

The following suggestions for oral care include many approaches as discussed in this text for conventional chemotherapy patients (see chapters 5, 7, 8). Attention here will be primarily directed at those situations unique to marrow transplantation.

Phase I

Patients being considered for transplantation should be examined for oral problems at the first possible opportunity. In the early years of marrow transplantation, patients were often in the end stages of their disease and comprehensive dental stabilization was not feasible. Now with patients in earlier stages of their malignancy it is possible to carry out more extensive dental treatment prior to transplant.

Following clinical and radiographic examination, all existing or potential sources of infection, trauma, or irritation should be eliminated. Scaling and dental prophylaxis should be carried out when possible. Deep carious lesions requiring immediate treatment should be repaired, as should sources of chronic irritation. It is important to remember that in some cases it may be as long as 10 to 12 months before subsequent restorative care can be reasonably considered. Furthermore, if a patient were to develop moderate to severe xerostomia for several months, initial decay could progress to become a significant problem, exposing the patient to possible systemic infection. The decision whether to begin endodontic therapy is potentially a critical choice since any foci of infection can spread to become potentially fatal. A recent study, however, indicates that asymptomatic pulpal pathosis may not require immediate endodontic therapy and acute pulpal infections without periapical involvement can be sufficiently resolved with initial endodontic therapy prior to myelosuppression without increased risk [53]. The question of how to treat symptomatic pulpal infections with periapical involvement is still unresolved. Nonrestorable or loose primary teeth are best extracted during Phase I. If partially erupted wisdom teeth are present, the potential for associated periodontal infections should be evaluated and treated accordingly. It is recommended that at least four to seven days be allowed for healing from surgical procedures before the start of chemoradiotherapy regimens. At least ten days of healing prior to onset of myelosuppression ($<1{,}000$ WBC/mm^3) is optimal. Partial and full dentures should function as atraumatically as possible and should be worn only when absolutely necessary. Orthodontic applicances are best removed because they are a major source of trauma, compromise oral hygiene, and increase the chance of infections.

Oral hygiene teaching and instructions should be given during Phase I and should cover brushing, flossing, and saline rinsing regimens. Adequate execution of these skills may strongly influence the severity of subsequent oral problems (see chapters 5,8).

Phase II

Parotid gland inflammation following total body radiation is best treated with ice packs and usually resolves in one to two days. Normal saline rinses are useful in facilitating expectoration of the viscous mucus saliva that follows radiation injury to the serous salivary gland acini. Frequent saline rinses and artificial salivas are useful for temporary relief of dryness. Salivary gland stimulants (pilocarpine 1%, sugarless lemon drops, or mints) can provide symptomatic relief by stimulating salivary flow until flow rates return to normal.

Management of mucositis generally is limited to the use of agents that reduce symptoms. A variety of topical pain-relief medications (anesthetics such as dyclonine, Xylocaine, diphenhydramine, and so on) are available and most are equally effective for managing moderate to severe stomatitis (see chapter 7). At times oral mucositis can become so severe that the only means available to control the pain are narcotic analgesics. Demerol, methadone, and morphine are employed depending on the patient's needs. Commercial mouthwashes (such as Cepacol and Chloraseptic) are best avoided. These solutions contain alcohol and phenol that dry and irritate damaged mucosa and can actually retard healing.

Oral infections should be treated aggressively with the appropriate systemic or topical antibiotics. Topical antibiotics, such as tetracycline, can be effective in some cases but systemic antibiotics are indicated if there is any sign of spread of infection or if the neutropenic patient becomes febrile [15,38]. A variety of topical antifungal agents are available. Nystatin, clotrimazole, and amphotericin B (topical) are used to control local infections while intravenous amphotericin B is used in invasive or systemic fungal infections. Acyclovir has helped reduce the frequency of severe viral stomatitis, but recurrent infections may be observed after stopping therapy.

Oral hemorrhage may be encountered when the patient is thrombocytopenic and can be both medically and psychologically disturbing. If moist-gauze pressure packs are not effective treatment, aggressive management with platelet transfusions and topical thrombin or microfibrillar collagen (Avitene) may be necessary. The clot can then be covered with

Orabase to protect the formed thrombus. Custom vinyl mouth guards might be useful for holding the topical hemostatic agent against the site of palatal or gingival bleeding and in preventing dislodgement of the clot. These devices can also be helpful in delivering other topical medications.

Phase III

It is important that patients continue to perform the intense oral hygiene regimens started earlier. Patients will begin to symptomatically improve and some will tend to discontinue all or most of the suggested care. Oral hygiene measures need to continue since immunologic and salivary recovery may take several more months. Fluoride treatments are recommended for both adults and children, especially when salivary flow rates are decreased [54].

The frequency of oral examinations will vary and depend on such factors as the severity of oral problems, compliance with oral hygiene regimens, and general medical status. Before each visit the patient's physician should be consulted and the current medical status reviewed. Personnel having direct contact with transplant patients should wear masks and gloves to minimize the chance of spreading infections to these immunologically compromised patients. Only dental work that is absolutely necessary should be attempted during this phase; it is recommended that work that can be postponed 8–12 months be delayed. Special attention should be directed toward detection of soft-tissue changes indicative of infection or chronic graft-versus-host disease. Oral labial biopsies have been safe and helpful in establishing the diagnosis of chronic graft-versus-host disease [42]. Prophylactic antibiotics are recommended for any invasive dental procedures, especially in patients with active chronic graft-versus-host disease.

Phase IV

Healthy long-term survivors without xerostomia can be managed essentially as normal dental patients. Patients who complain of xerostomia or who have demonstrated decreased salivary flow rates must be monitored carefully for compliance with oral hygiene measures. Furthermore, they should be provided with topical fluoride and custom vinyl trays and given instruction in the daily use of fluoride treatments. Patients with active chronic graft-versus-host disease who are receiving immunosuppressive and prophylactic antibiotic therapy are similar to patients in earlier phases where immune function may be significantly compromised. The exact oral regimens will be determined by the type and extent of oral involvement. Careful planning and frequent follow-up is especially important where chronic graft-versus-host disease involvement is severe and oral tissues are atrophic, inflamed, and friable. Currently the topical use of steroids for oral chronic graft-versus-host disease is of uncertain usefulness, and oral improvement is generally dependent on the response to systemic regimens [27]. Antifungal medications are beneficial to reduce the influence of low-level candidal infections.

The oral cavity may have a profound psychological impact on the transplant patient. Oral problems can be among the most frequent and severe causes of morbidity on the transplant ward. Oral pain and bleeding can be extremely discomforting. Patient education can reduce anxiety and increase treatment compliance. It is not surprising, therefore, that effective care of oral complications can be one of the most appreciated and remembered interactions for the marrow transplant recipient.

SUMMARY

Once considered a desperate form of therapy for end-stage patients, bone-marrow transplantation is now considered effective treatment for severe aplastic anemia, acute leukemia, and immunodeficiency disease. Marrow transplantation is a complex and challenging procedure that requires the expertise of teams of individuals utilizing their specific knowledge of clinical medicine and basic science.

Marrow may be obtained from the patient (autologous) or from family members (allogeneic or syngeneic transplant). Supralethal total body irradiation and/or high-dose chemotherapy are used to destroy the patient's own bone marrow, eliminate any malignant cells, and/or prevent graft rejection. Hematologic engraftment and recovery is from cells of donor origin and is noted 20–30 days after marrow infusion. Full immunologic reconstitution, however, may require many more months. The oral cavity is frequently a site of severe complications. Following marrow ablation, patients are susceptible to a variety of oral viral, bacterial, and fungal infections, bleeding, severe mucositis, and xerostomia. These problems cause significant morbidity and can be potentially life-threatening. In addition, chronic graft-versus-host disease is an autoimmune-like disorder that may develop following engraftment. Oral involvement with chronic graft-versus-host disease includes atrophic mucositis, a Sjögren's-like xerostomia, and a variety of mucocutaneous changes that can mimic such diseases as lichen planus, lupus erythematosus, and scleroderma. Oral care and management of complications plays an important part in successful bone-marrow transplantation.

REFERENCES

1. Jacobson LO, Simmons EL, Marks EK, et al.: The role of the spleen in radiation injury and recovery. J Lab Clin Med (35):746–770, 1950.
2. Lorenz E, Uphoff D, Reid TR, Shelton E: Modification of irradiation injury in mice and guinea pigs by bone marrow injections. J Natl Cancer Inst (12):197–201, 1951.
3. Thomas ED, Lochte HL Jr, Lu WC, Ferrebee JW: Intravenous infusion of bone marrow in patients receiving radiation and chemotherapy. N Engl J Med (257):491–496, 1957.
4. Camitta BM, Thomas ED, Nathan DG, Gale RP, Kopecky KJ, Rapport JM, Santos G, Gordon-Smith EC, Storb R: A prospective study of androgens and bone marrow transplantation for treatment of severe aplastic anemia. Blood (53):504–514, 1979.
5. Storb R, Doney KC, Thomas ED, Appelbaum F, Buckner CD, Clift RA: Marrow transplantation with or without buffy coat cells for 65 transfused aplastic anemia patients. Blood (59):236–246, 1982.
6. Storb R, Thomas ED, Buckner CD, Clift RA, Deeg HS, Fefer A, Goodell RW, Sale GE, Sanders J, Singer J, Stewart P, Weiden PL: Marrow transplantation in thirty "untransfused" patients with severe aplastic anemia. Ann Intern Med (92):30–36, 1980.
7. Thomas ED, Buckner ED, Clift RA, Fefer A, Johnson FL, Neiman PE, Sale GE, Sanders JE, Singer JW, Shulman H, Storb R, Weiden PL: Marrow transplantation for acute nonlymphoblastic leukemia in first remission. N Engl J Med (301):597–599, 1979.
8. Fefer A, Cheever MA, Greenberg PD, Appelbaum FR, Boyd W, Buckner CD, et al.: Treatment of chronic granulocytic leukemia with chemoradiotherapy and transplantation of marrow from identical twins. N Engl J Med (306):63–68, 1982.
9. Hansen JA, Clift RA, Thomas ED, Buckner CD, Storb R, Giblett ER: Transplantation of marrow from an unrelated donor to a patient with acute leukemia. N Engl J Med (303):565–567, 1980.
10. Thomas DE: Bone marrow transplantation: Present status and future expectations. In *Update I; Harrison's Principles of Internal Medicine,* Issenbach KJ, Adams RA, Braunwald E, Martin JB, Petersdorf RG, Wilson JD (eds), New York, McGraw-Hill, 1981.

11. Appelbaum FR, Fefer A, Cheever MA, Sanders JE, Singer JW, Adamson JW, Mickelson EM, Hansen JA, Greenberg PD, Thomas ED: Treatment of aplastic anemia by bone marrow transplantation in identical twins. Blood (55):1033–1039, 1980.
12. Clift RA, Hansen JA, Thomas ED: The role of HLA in marrow transplantation. Transplant Proc (13):-234–236, 1981.
13. Thomas ED, Storb R, Clift RA, Fefer A, Johnson FL, Neiman PE, Lerner KG, Glucksberg H, Buckner CD: Bone marrow transplantation. N Engl J Med (292):832–843, 895–902, 1975.
14. Neiman P, Thomas ED, Buckner CD, Storb R, Fefer A, Glucksberg H, Lerner KG: Marrow transplantation for aplastic anemia and acute leukemia. Ann Rev Med (25):179–198, 1974.
15. Meyers JD, Thomas ED: Infection complicating bone marrow transplantation. In *Clinical Approach to Infection in the Immunocompromised Host,* Young LS, Rubin RH (eds), New York, Plenum, 1981.
16. Buckner CD, Clift RA, Sanders JE, Meyers JD, Counts GW, Farewell VT, Thomas ED: Protective environment for marrow transplant recipients. A prospective study. Ann Int Med (89):893–901, 1978.
17. Clift RA, Sanders JE, Thomas ED, Williams B, Buckner CD: Granulocyte transfusions for the prevention of infection in patients receiving bone marrow transplants. N Engl J Med (298):1052–1057, 1978.
18. Saral R, Burns WH, Laskin DL, Santos GW, Lietman P: Acyclovir prophylaxis of herpes simplex infections: A randomized, double blind, controlled trial in bone marrow transplant recipients. N Engl J Med (305):63–67, 1981.
19. Hickman RO, Buckner CO, Clift RA, Sanders JE, Stewart P, Thomas ED: A modified right arterial catheter for access to the venous system in marrow transplant recipients. Surg Gynecol Obstet (148):871–875, 1979.
20. Storb R: Bone marrow transplantation for the treatment of hematologic malignancy and of aplastic anemia. Transplant Proc (13):221–226, 1981.
21. Slavin RE, Santos GW: The graft-versus-host reaction in man after bone marrow transplantation: Pathology, pathogenesis, clinical features and implications. Clin Immunol Immunopathol (1):472–498, 1973.
22. Glucksberg H, Storb R, Fefer A, Buckner CD, Neiman PE, Clift RA, Lerner KG, Thomas ED; Clinical manifestations of graft-versus-host disease in human recipients of marrow from HLA matched sibling donors. Transplantation (18):295–304, 1974.
23. Shulman HM, Sullivan KM, Weiden PL, McDonald GB, Striker GE, Sale GE, Hackman R, Tsoi MS, Storb R, Thomas ED: Chronic graft-versus-host syndrome in man. A long term clinicopathologic study of 20 Seattle patients. Am J Med (69):204–217, 1982.
24. Atkinson K, Storb R, Prentice RL, Weiden P, Witherspoon RP, Sullivan KM, Noel D, Thomas ED: Analysis of late infections in 89 long term survivors of bone marrow transplantation. Blood (53):720–731, 1979.
25. Powles RL, Clink HM, Spence D, Morgenstern G, Watson JG, Selby PJ, Woods M, Barrett A, Jameson B, Sloane J, Lawler SD, Kay H, Lawson D, McElwain T, Alexander P: Cyclosporin A to prevent graft-versus-host disease in man after allogeneic bone marrow transplantation. Lancet (8164):327–329, 1980.
26. Weiden PL, Fluornoy N, Sanders JF, Sullivan KM, Thomas ED: Antileukemic effect of graft-versus-host disease contributes to improved survival after allogeneic marrow transplantation. Transplant Proc (12):-248–251, 1981.
27. Sullivan KM, Shulman HM, Storb R, Weider PL, Witherspoon RP, McDonald GB, Schubert MM, Atkinson K, Thomas ED: Chronic graft-versus-host disease in 52 patients: Adverse natural course and successful treatment with combination immunosuppression. Blood (57):267–276, 1981.
28. Witherspoon RP, Kopecky K, Storb RF, Fluornoy N, Sullivan KM, Sosa R, Deeg HJ, Ochs HD, Cheevers MA, Fefer A, Thomas ED: Immunological recovery in 48 patients following syngeneic marrow transplantation for hematological malignancy. Transplantation (33):143–149, 1982.
29. Witherspoon RP, Storb R, Ochs Hd, Flournoy N, Kopecky K, Sullivan KM, Deeg HJ, Sosa R, Noel DR, Atkinson K, Thomas ED: Recovery of antibody production in human allogeneic marrow graft recipients: Influence of time post transplantation, the presence or absence of chronic graft-versus-host disease, and antithymocyte globulin treatment. Blood (58):360–368, 1981.
30. Tsoi MS, Storb R, Dobbs S, Kopecky KJ, Santos E, Weiden PL, Thomas ED: Nonspecific suppressor cells in patients with chronic graft-versus-host disease after marrow grafting. J Immunol (123):1970–1976, 1979.
31. Tsoi MS, Storb R, Dobb S, Thomas ED: Specific suppressor cells in graft-host tolerance of HLA-identical marrow transplantation. Nature (292):355–357, 1981.
32. Lockhart PB, Sonis ST: Relationship of oral complications to peripheral blood leukocyte and platelet counts in patients receiving cancer chemotherapy. Oral Surg (48):21–28, 1979.
33. Dreizen S, Bodey GP, Rodriquez V: Oral complications of cancer chemotherapy. Postgrad Med (58):75–82, 1975.
34. Silverman S: Radiation effects. In *Oral Cancer,* Silverman S (ed), New York, American Cancer Society, 1981.
35. Dreizen S: Stomatotoxic manifestations of cancer chemotherapy. J Prosthet Dent (40):650–655, 1978.
36. Gershwin ME, Goetzl EJ, Steinberg AD: Cyclophosphamide: Use in practice. Ann Intern Med (80):531–540, 1974.

37. Chabner BA, Myers CE, Coleman CN, Johns DG: The clinical pharmacology of antineoplastic agents. N Engl J Med (292):1107–1113, 1159–1168, 1975.
38. Dreizen S, Bodey GP, Brown LR: Opportunistic gram-negative bacillary infections in leukemia—oral manifestations during myelosuppression. Postgrad Med (55):133–139, 1974.
39. Solberg CO, Meuwissen HJ, Needham RN, Good RA, Matsen JM: Infectious complications in bone marrow transplant patients. Br Med J (1):18–23, 1971.
40. Dreizen S, McCredie KB, Sicke KA, Zander AR, Peters JL: Oral complications of bone marrow transplantation in adults with acute leukemia. Postgrad Med (66):187–194, 1979.
41. Morris PG: Cyclosporin A: Overview. Transplantation (32):349–354, 1981.
42. Schubert MM, Truelove EL, Sullivan KM, Izutsu KT, Flournoy N, Kolbinson DA: Oral signs of chronic graft-versus-host disease. Proc J Dent Res (68):263, 1982.
43. Sale GE, Shulman HM, Schubert MM, Sullivan KM, Kopecky KJ, Hackman RC, Morton TH, Storb R, Thomas ED: Oral and opthalmic pathology of graft versus host disease in man: Predictive value of the lips biopsy. Hum Pathol (12):1022–1030, 1981.
44. Gratwohl AA, Moutsopoulos HM, Chused TM, Akizuki M, Wolf RO, Sweet JB, Reisseroth AB: Sjögren-type syndrome after allogeneic bone marrow transplantation. Ann Intern Med 87:703–706, 1977.
45. Mandel ID, Burmash H: Sialochemistry in Sjögren's syndrome. Oral Surg, Oral Med, Oral Pathol (41): 182–187, 1976.
46. Moutsopoulous H, Karsh J, Wolf R, Tarpley T: Lysozyme determination in parotid saliva from patients with Sjögren's syndrome. Am J Med (69):39–42, 1980.
47. Izutsu K, Oberg S, Shulman H, Schubert M, Sullivan K, Morton T, Sale G, Truelove E: Depressed salivary IgA; and sodium and flow changes in C-GVHD patients. J Supramol Struct (Suppl A):24, 1980.
48. Izutsu KT, Schubert MM, Shulman H, Oberg S, Sullivan KM, Rice J, Morton T, Truelove E: Salivary changes in graft-versus-host disease (GVHD) Proc J Dent Res (95–A): 401, 1980.
49. Izutsu KT, Truelove EL, Schubert MM, Ensign WY, Meadows EE: Does graft-versus-host disease cause hyposalivation in bone marrow transplant recipients? Proc J Dent Res (68):263, 1982.
50. Truelove EL, Izutsu KT, Schubert MM, Ensign WT, Meadows EE: Salivary lysozyme levels are increased in bone marrow transplant (BMT) recipients. Proc J Dent Res (68):223, 1982.
51. Izutsu KT, Schubert MM, Truelove EL, Shulman HM, Sale GE, Morton TH, Ensign WY, Mersai T, Thomas DE: The predictive value of elevated sodium concentration: Its relation to labial gland pathology in bone marrow transplant recipients. Hum Pathol (May 1982, in press).
52. Beschorner WE, Yardley JH, Tutschka PJ, Santos GW: Deficiency of intestinal immunity with graft-versus-host disease in humans. J Infect Dis (144):38–46, 1981.
53. Peterson DE, Overholser CD, Williams LT: Endodontic therapy in patients receiving myelosuppressive chemotherapy. Proc J Dent Res (61):276, 1982.
54. Rakocz M, Serota FT, Nelson LP, Reich DR, Werther PL, August CS: Dental management of the child undergoing bone marrow transplantation, JADA (104):485–488, 1982.

7. DENTAL MANAGEMENT OF PATIENTS RECEIVING CHEMOTHERAPY

PETER B. LOCKHART, D.D.S.

INTRODUCTION

The diagnosis and management of oral complications of cancer therapy often provide difficult challenges in the area of oral medicine. Because of the increased incidence, severity, and duration of these problems and the potential threat to patient survival, they must be evaluated and managed in the most thorough manner. Although most oral disease is managed with a surgical as opposed to medical approach, cancer patients frequently manifest their oral problems at a point in their therapy when surgical manipulation of any type is contraindicated. These patients therefore must often be managed medically until more definitive treatment can be performed. Furthermore, the surgical treatment itself is frequently the most straightforward aspect of the overall oral management. The actual diagnosis, timing, and modifications in methods of treatment are often the most difficult aspects in the care of these patients.

Ideally, all patients about to undergo cancer chemotherapy should first be thoroughly evaluated by a general dentist with expertise in this field. The nature and scope of oral problems encountered in this patient population draws on the multidisciplinary background of the generalist who can offer the necessary range of treatment [1]. There may not be sufficient time for elective therapy, but the history, exam, and radiographs provide a baseline that may be helpful should problems subsequently arise.

PRETREATMENT EVALUATION

Paramount to the overall dental management of cancer patients is the pretreatment evaluation. Prior to the initial patient visit, it is necessary to have a thorough understanding of

D.E. Peterson and S.T. Sonis (eds.), ORAL COMPLICATIONS OF CANCER CHEMOTHERAPY, 113-149.

the patient's overall medical status and any plans for cancer therapy (table 7–1). These factors will largely determine what dental treatment, if any, can be accomplished at this time. Any additional information about the patient, including social and family history, is useful for overall evaluation.

Present oral complaint

Many patients are seen for a specific oral problem at some point in their cancer therapy. The patient's own story is often critical to an assessment of his or her problem, since radiographs and other diagnostic procedures may not be feasible on a nonambulatory patient, and the oral picture may be altered by immunosuppression. Allow the patient to relate the problem from its inception to the present time. The onset, timing, severity, character, and course of the problem should be noted in order to differentiate between such pathoses as pulpal versus periodontal, temperomandibular joint versus odontogenic,

Table 7–1. Pretreatment Evaluation

Review recent medical history.

Present oral complaint
- Onset, timing, severity, character, and course of the problem
- Degree of limitation
- Medications used past and present
- Exacerbated by, relieved by

Past dental history
- Frequency of past visits, including hygiene
- History of extractions, periodontal surgery, endodontics, pain, swelling, bleeding, ulcers
- Home care: hygiene methods
- Diet

Oral examination
- Extraoral
  - Observe for limited movement, speech changes, asymmetries.
  - Palpate for nodes, swellings, tenderness.
- Intraoral
  - Remove appliances: examine for fit, function, and aesthetics.
  - With gloves, tongue blade, light, and mirror:

Examine:	labial mucosa	*For:*	color changes	*Note:*	appearance
	buccal mucosa		lesions		location
	floor of mouth		swelling		size
	palate		bleeding		shape
	pharynx		plaques		depth
	tongue		infection		number
	gingiva		xerostomia		degree
			texture		

  - Examine teeth for plaque, calculus, caries, mobility, faulty restorations, fractures.

Radiographs
- Full series desirable (panorex and bitewings alternative)
- Examine for bone loss, caries, root tips, impactions, calculus, periapical/furcation radiolucencies, fractures.

Laboratory values
- WBC + differential, platelet count
- PT, PTT, Bleeding time
- Blood cultures

or benign ulcerative versus invasive infectious phenomena. The patient's manner in relating a problem may give insight into the overall effect it is having on their status. For example, the need for topical or systemic pain medications and the need for dietary supplements or artificial feeding can often be determined at this point in the patient evaluation.

The detail of this aspect of the history will be predicated on several factors such as the degree of patient debilitation and the complexity of the problem and its management. However, the diagnosis can often be made with some certainty on the basis of the medical history and the patient description alone.

Past dental history

Patients are surprisingly receptive to dental history taking when they first understand both the nature of the problems that can result from their cancer therapy and the importance of measures to prevent these morbidities. Depending on the reason for the dental evaluation, a complete past dental history may or may not be of value. Nevertheless, there is some dental historical data that is important in the evaluation and treatment planning of these patients (table 7–1.).

The frequency of past dental visits, including hygiene and any history of extractions, periodontal surgery, and endodontics gives the clinician an indication of the degree of dental awareness and motivation. A patient whose past dental visits were essentially crisis-oriented may be treatment planned very differently from a patient who has always had routine dental care by a general dentist. Patients should be questioned concerning their usual diet, frequency of brushing and flossing, and use of any other hygiene measures. Any history of oral or maxillofacial pain, swelling, bleeding, or other oral problems should be developed. This data base should give the clinician a reasonable understanding of the patient's past dental history and provide clues for further questioning. The patient may relate subtle symptoms of existing or potential problems that may worsen significantly following chemotherapy. Patients who have already received chemotherapy should be questioned in some detail concerning any oral problems that were experienced. Lastly, some idea as to the need for patient education will develop during the course of the patient interview.

Oral examination

The examination of these patients is often done under far less than ideal circumstances. The patient may be debilitated, in considerable oral pain, have limited oral opening, and have debris or medications that obscure the mucosa. In spite of these handicaps, every effort should be made to thoroughly evaluate the hard and soft oral tissues. Needless to say, the extent of the oral exam depends largely on the reason for the exam and the ability of the patient to tolerate it. Care must be exercised, as innocuous-appearing lesions can be acutely painful. In addition, since a repeat exam may need to be done on a daily basis, the trust and cooperation of the patient is critical. The use of topical anaesthetics prior to the exam may be helpful in some cases. The clinician must always remain empathetic to the intense discomfort some patients endure with their mouths and be skilled in an oral exam that will give the necessary information to assess the problem.

Extraoral exam

Much information concerning the patient's oral status can be gathered by close observation of the patient during the history-taking aspect of the workup. The patient's affect, degree of oral discomfort, xerostomia and other limitations are often readily apparent. Observe the patient for extraoral facial and labial lesions (for example, herpetiform) and asymmetries or swellings. Following this, with clean hands or gloves, palpate the head and neck region for lymph nodes (noting the submental, submandibular, and cervical chain areas). Palpate the facial muscles and buccal and labial areas for indication of oral discomfort and the need for care in the intraoral examination.

Intraoral exam

Any intraoral examination of the patient should be done with well-scrubbed hands or sterile gloves to protect against possible hospital-acquired infectious organisms. Clinicians and others working around the patient's mouth should be aware of the greater potential for hepatitis transmission due to the large number of transfusions necessary in this group of patients. Therefore gloves and masks should be worn when carrying out any procedures that involve contact with saliva [2].

Have the patient remove any appliances from the mouth for examination (table 7–1). Gently lift the upper and lower lips away from the teeth. With a bright flashlight or headlamp examine the labial mucosa for color changes, abrasions, ulcerations, swellings, plaques, or bleeding. At the same time, examine the gingiva for color, size, texture, consistency, and contour. Observe for evidence of gingival bleeding or infection. With wet tongue depressors (and a mirror, if needed) examine the buccal mucosa, floor of mouth, all surfaces of the tongue and palate (anterior to posterior) and as much of the pharyngeal wall as can be visualized. Any changes from normal should be noted, paying particular attention to color, coatings, lesions, and evidence of infection or bleeding, and noting carefully the appearance, size, and location of each. Much can be learned about a patient's overall systemic status by careful observation of the oral soft tissues. If a base-line exam has been carefully documented, the degree and the rate of change of the mucosal tissues often heralds or mirrors changes in the patient's marrow or clinical status.

Following this, examine the teeth for deposits (plaque and calculus), caries, and state of any existing resotrations. Mobility of any teeth should be noted. The gingiva should be palpated and the teeth lightly percussed with a tongue blade. More involved thermal and electrical testing can be deferred unless needed in the evaluation of the neurovascular status of specific teeth. Probing of periodontal pockets is difficult outside the dental operatory and in the absence of good lighting. In addition, probing or other elective gingival manipulation should not be done on severely neutropenic patients.

Removable appliances should be evaluated for fit, esthetics, function, and overall need for use; instructions on the use of such appliances can be critical during certain phases of treatment.

The use of intraoral photography to document the size, location, and coloration of oral lesions is often helpful in determining the degree of progression or regression of oral mucosal alterations.

Radiographs

Whenever possible, a full-mouth series of radiographs should be obtained. However, this step may need to be deferred if the patient is too ill to be transported or to tolerate such an evaluation or has little in the history or exam to suggest an odontogenic problem. Much essential information on the patient's oral status can be gained from periapical and bitewing films of the teeth and supporting structures. Asymptomatic patients are often found on radiographic exam to have dental disease that could become life-threatening, if not simply troublesome, once the patient becomes myelosuppressed. Horizontal and vertical alveolar bone loss, retained root tips, deep caries, and periapical pathoses can often only be visualized on good intraoral radiographs. Panoramic and other extraoral radiographs can be helpful if intraoral films cannot be obtained but usually offer only a general overview of the jaws and teeth. An attempt should be made, when indicated, to obtain any preexisting dental radiographs and other relevant information from the patient's dentist. This previous information may be compared to the present condition or may eliminate the need for taking films on a compromised patient.

Laboratory values

The most important laboratory values in the assessment of these patients are the total white blood count and differential (notably the polymorphonuclear leukocytes, lymphocytes, and blast forms) and the platelet count. Other values such as the bleeding, prothrombin, and partial thromboplastin time and other clotting parameters may be important if contemplating surgical treatment or evaluating a bleeding problem. Care must be exercised in the interpretation of these values as they may change significantly in a 24-hour period and may merely represent quantitative values and not the qualitative status of the platelet or white blood cell (WBC).

Those individuals who come in contact with saliva should be aware of the increased exposure these patients have to hepatitis from repeated transfusion of blood products. Since time and circumstances usually preclude the evaluation of this possibility, these patients should be managed with this in mind.

TREATMENT PLANNING

Often the most difficult dental decisions to be made on these patients are those concerning the type, timing, and aggressiveness of therapy to be performed. Once the history, exam, and necessary diagnostic data have been gathered, a plan often must be formulated on short notice. A major determinant in treatment planning is the patient's marrow status at the time and what will happen to the peripheral blood counts within the next seven to ten days. Various treatment modifications are discussed in later sections with reference to marrow status and myelosuppression.

The widely held past philosophy that all patients should have all of their teeth extracted prior to treatment is no longer valid [3,4]. Careful treatment planning and therapy can create a situation where odontogenic infection is highly unlikely without the needless physical and psychological trauma from the removal of teeth. Hopeless teeth, however, should be extracted. Scaling and curretage should leave the remaining teeth clean of any supra- and subgingival deposits. The periodontal pocket depths should be measured with consideration for the shrinkage that may occur following healing from the oral prophylaxis. Teeth with pockets greater than 4–5 mm should be evaluated carefully with regard to the patient's ability to keep them plaque-free and the potential for problems later when any invasive therapy is contraindicated. These considerations are especially important with molar teeth due to the problem of maintaining root furcation involvements disease-free. In addition, the age of the patient, degree of motivation, and overall medical prognosis are important factors in decisions to maintain teeth. Following this, attention can be directed at the adequacy of existing restorations and appliances. Sharp teeth and appliances should be recontoured and polished (figure 7–1). Teeth with old or defective restorations should be evaluated for evidence of pulp necrosis. Large amalgam (in posterior teeth) and composite (in anterior teeth) restorations are often indicated as alternatives to crowns. Appliances should be tightened, relined, or otherwise adjusted to fit and function well without exerting stress or friction on supporting hard and soft tissues. It should be kept in mind that aesthetics and function are no less important to these patients and they in fact may become obsessed with these factors. Every effort should be made to provide an aesthetic, functional, comfortable, and disease-free mouth.

PREVENTIVE THERAPY

There is a strong feeling among dentists caring for these patients that the prechemotherapy oral status—in particular, the presence of caries and/or periodontal disease—greatly influences the incidence of morbidities following cancer chemotherapy. Prevention of many of these oral complications is therefore not only possible but essential in the comprehensive management of these patients (table 7–2.).

Patient education

One advantage of early involvement of dentistry in the overall management of cancer patients is the opportunity to discuss oral problems that can occur during therapy. Many patients become highly motivated in mouth care once they realize the role of the mouth as a possible cause of problems distant from the mouth and the active role the patient can play in the prevention of these problems. Patients usually welcome the opportunity to become actively involved in their own care. An occasional patient may even have to be cautioned against overzealous brushing or flossing in order to keep mouth care itself from initiating or prolonging a problem.

Once patients understand the rationale for scrupulous hygiene they should be instructed in oral hygiene methods and aids for their particular situation. The dental hygienist, if available, is an excellent resource for help in this endeavor. In addition, the patient's nurse(s) should also become actively involved as she/he spends large amounts of time with the patient and can supervise, and carry out when necessary, the indicated hygiene measures [5].

Hygiene/appliances

Hygiene measures recommended for the patient are varied and depend greatly on the patient's level of myelosuppression and ability to tolerate soft-tissue manipulation. As

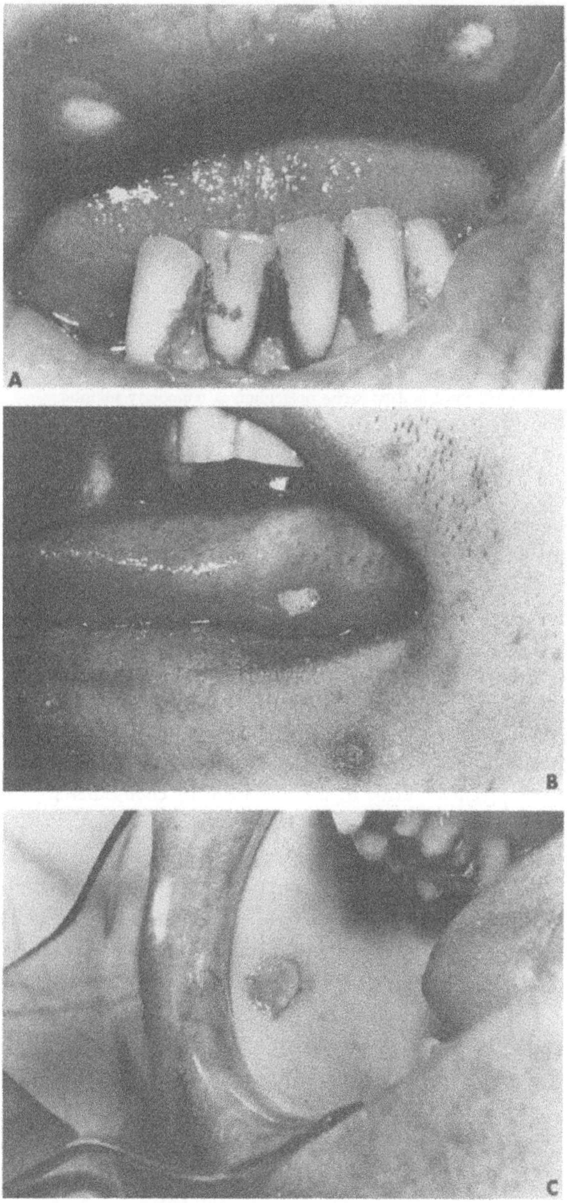

Figure 7–1.

A. 38-year-old neutropenic patient on chemotherapy for leukemia. Note secondarily infected ulcerations which originated from sharp mandibular anterior teeth.

B. 25-year-old leukemic patient with WBC = 150/mm^3. Note moderately deep, secondarily infected ulceration on the lateral border of the tongue, and moderate swelling in absence of neutrophils. This is a common location for trauma from teeth.

C. 45-year-old neutropenic patient with lymphoma. Note shallow, superficially infected ulceration without surrounding erythema that was caused by trauma from the adjacent teeth.

Table 7-2 General Principles of Prevention

Patient and staff education
Meticulous oral hygiene
Professional cleaning if possible and blood counts permit
Do not discontinue with administration of chemotherapy, continue until neutropenic or clinical intolerance (bleeding, pain, low counts, et cetera) then switch to gauze cleaning (wet 2×2 wrapped around finger).
H_2O_2–H_2O–mouthwash (1:1:1) rinses several times/day; discontinue mouthwash or H_2O_2 if it irritates mucosa.
Eliminate all sources of irritation.
Remove all oral appliances including orthodontic retainers and bands and leave out with onset of myelosuppression.
Eliminate sharp teeth by smoothing or extraction.
Eliminate potential sources of infection
Remove overhanging margins on crowns, restorations, and so on.
Extract questionable teeth (caries, periodontally involved).
Extract partially erupted third molars; excise operculum as temporary solution.
Apply vaseline to dry, cracked lips.
Antifungal therapy
Nystatin 100,000 U swish and swallow qid; when WBC begins to drop, increase to 300,000 U qid.
Nystatin lozenges if needed for prolonged contact with mucosa
+ barium swallow → amphotericin B
Increase resistance to xerostomia-induced caries
meticulous oral hygiene
fluoride rinses qd
artificial saliva
frequent professional cleanings

mentioned earlier, absolute numbers of circulating blood cells are helpful but not all inclusive in determining the degree of myelosuppression. The patient's disease itself may predispose to oral problems prior to the initiation of chemotherapy [6,7].

As the patient's blood counts begin to drop following chemotherapy, hygiene measures should be adjusted accordingly. In the absence of well-controlled studies—either animal or human—it is difficult to know at what point certain hygiene measures should be dropped or modified. However, studies are presently being conducted to resolve this dilemma. Oral hygiene is an attempt to prevent localized infection such as gingivitis or periodontitis from exacerbating during chemotherapy. Such an exacerbation can result in fever and life-threatening, if not debilitating, maxillofacial or distant infection. Balanced against this is the threat that routine oral hygiene measures themselves may seed organisms into the systemic circulation through the gingival crevice and infect a distant site or organ.

Prechemotherapy

Hygiene measures at times when the patient is not severely myelosuppressed (WBC > $2000/mm^3$ with > 20% polymorphonuclear leukocytes, and platelets > $20{,}000/mm^3$) should be aggressive and closely monitored. A thorough scaling and prophylaxis is ideal when possible. Brushing (soft brush) and flossing should be carried out at least daily, under supervision in the beginning, ideally at night after the last meal of the day. Rinsing with sterile saline or water several times a day is helpful, especially after meals, to debride the teeth and lower the bacterial and acid level in the mouth. Appliances can be worn if the patient desires as long as the soft tissues are monitored for irritation or ulcer formation.

Loose-fitting dentures or partials can be soft-relined on a temporary basis until more ideal adjustments can be accomplished.

During myelosuppression

It is the feeling of many dentists involved with these patients that when the patient's total white blood counts drop below 1,500–2,000/mm^3 with less than 10% polymorphonuclear leukocytes, brushing and flossing should be stopped. This is a controversial subject and each patient should be considered individually as there are no absolute guidelines on safe and unsafe peripheral blood counts. The threat of bacteremia from oral hygiene measures must be weighed against the risk of progressive gingival disease and resultant bacteremias that can occur through the ulcerated gingival crevice [8]. Patients may be too debilitated at this point in their treatment to do much more for themselves than mouth rinsing. They can be instructed in the use of wet 2×2 or 4×4 sponges wrapped around an index finger to debride the teeth, gingiva, and tongue, and to use frequent (every two to four hours) and vigorous mouth rinses, especially after eating. Oral irrigation devices are of limited value in that they may only remove gross debris and have been reported to cause bacteremias in nonimmunosuppressed patients [9]. Many patients are unable to carry out mouth care themselves and should have this done for them. With proper patient positioning to avoid choking or aspiration, the dentist, nurse, or hygienist can then irrigate and suction the mouth with a large syringe or inverted enema bag (see chapter 8). Patients with severe mucositis and tissue sloughing may benefit from careful irrigation as often as every two hours.

Oral bleeding is another common problem associated with myelosuppression. As noted, the absolute number of platelets is not the sole determinant of the patient's propensity for bleeding. Some patients may experience spontaneous submucosal or gingival bleeding with $> 30,000$ platelets/mm^3 while others may be free of spontaneous bleeding at $< 1,000$/mm^3 (figure 7–2). As a general rule, the incidence of oral bleeding increases almost exponentially with platelet counts below 20,000/mm^3, and more care should be exercised with hygiene measures [10]. If other blood counts permit, brushing and flossing can be continued well below 20,000/mm^3 but should be stopped in favor of rinses if bleeding occurs with brushing. Once again, the patient may be faced with the cyclic problem of decreased hygiene leading to an increase in plaque, inflammation, and potential for gingival bleeding (figure 7–3). Most patients, however, who are troubled with gingival bleeding may be made worse with any undue trauma to these tissues.

The recommendations just given apply to the use of intraoral removable appliances as well. Appliances that have less than ideal fit as a result of wear or weight loss can traumatize the fragile oral mucosa (figure 7–4). In addition, bacteremias can be generated from torque forces on the supporting teeth. With inadequate hygiene, appliances can serve as a reservoir for growth of pathogenic bacteria and fungi. Therefore, once the blood counts begin to decrease, oral appliances should be left out of the mouth until the patient is beyond the point of concern for bleeding and bacteremia. On occasion, whether for psychological or nutritional purposes, these restrictions may be lifted for short periods, but the patient should be closely monitored to insure that appliance-related problems do not occur.

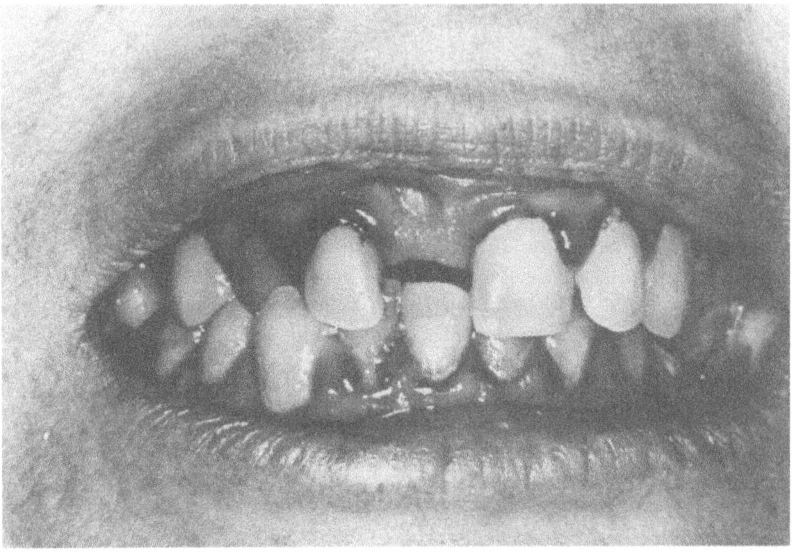

Figure 7–2. 49-year-old pancytopenic woman with a total platelet count of 800/mm³. Note hematoma formation at gingival crest around all teeth but absence of spontaneous bleeding in spite of local irritants and severe thrombocytopenia.

Fluoride

Fluoride has long been known to be of significant benefit in the prevention of caries. Therefore, patients with active carious lesions, regardless of size, should be put on a daily fluoride rinse. Patients often receive chemotherapy before even temporary restorative dental treatment can be accomplished, and a combination of scrupulous hygiene, low sugar intake, and fluoride rinses may significantly decrease the possibility of an acute pulpitis and subsequent alveolar abscess. Fluoride is known to prevent colonization of bacteria around teeth [11] and to have bacteriostatic effects, but this has not yet been studied in this patient population. Nevertheless, in a situation where the oral flora has such devastating potential, and efforts to sterilize the oral cavity have been disappointing [12], the use of fluoride may be of significant benefit.

Patients should be supervised initially in their use of fluoride and ideally be able to rinse for one to two minutes and expectorate, not swallow, the solution. This is best carried out after the last meal of the day and following routine oral hygiene measures. Should an acidulated fluoride rinse stimulate painful mucosa, a nonacidulated form can be utilized.

EVALUATION AND MANAGEMENT CONSIDERATIONS

Diet

Nutrition often becomes a particularly difficult problem for these patients. Many of the cancer therapies and their sequelae predispose patients to xerostomia, pain, loss of taste and appetite, nausea and general debilitation, all of which detract from adequate nutrition.

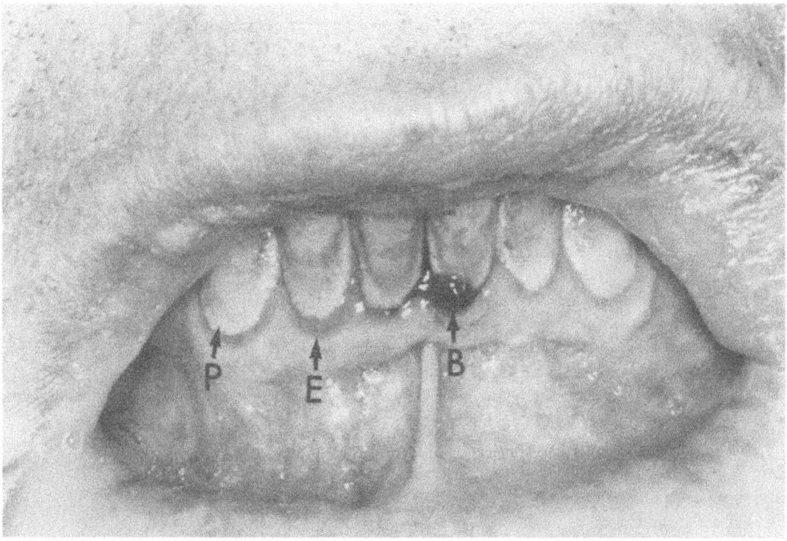

Figure 7–3. 53-year-old male with aplastic anemia and chronic thrombocytopenia. Note local irritants of plaque *(P)* and calculus and the erythema *(E)* and spontaneous bleeding *(B)* that results. With adequate platelet coverage, a thorough scaling resolved the acute gingival disease and the spontaneous bleeding ceased.

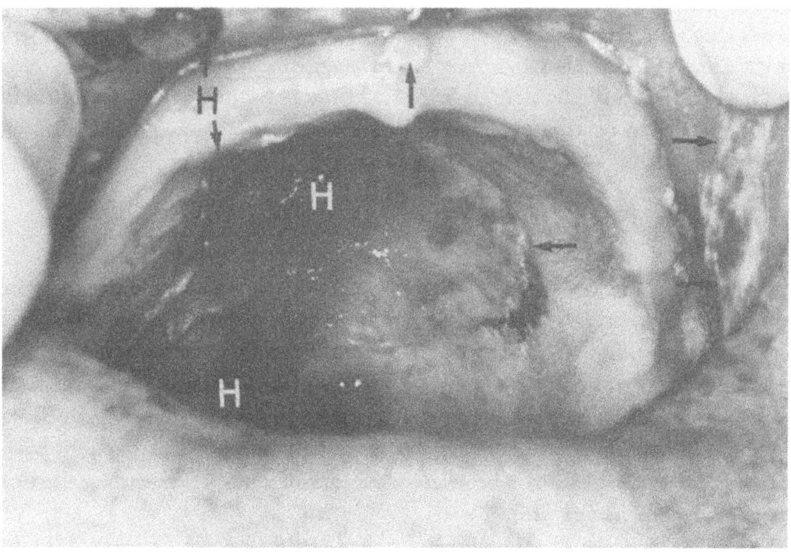

Figure 7–4. 53-year-old male one week from methotrexate chemotherapy. Note severe maxillary mucosal ulcerations and hemorrhage *(H)* which resulted from 24 hour/day denture use. Ulcers correspond to denture flanges and areas of tissue pressure *(arrows)*.

Table 7–3 Dietary measures for patients receiving cancer chemotherapy

For problems of
Xerostomia, mucositis, ulcers, sore throat
Reduce discomfort by
Avoiding rough foods that can injure mucosa (for example, toast)
Choosing soft or liquid foods
Trying melted margarine, gravy, broth, cream, or cheese sauce to moisten foods
Using foods softened or moistened by dipping in coffee, tea, milk, broth, or swallowing beverage with bite of food
Trying strained beef, pork, chicken, or fish for protein
Mashing potatoes and straining vegetables
Mashing fruits such as bananas, pears, peaches
Eating cool or room-temperature foods (ice cream, sherbet, popsicles, watermelon, yogurt, custard)
Trying chicken, beef, or vegetable soups
Using sugarless candy or mints to stimulate saliva production
Drinking warm tea, coffee, cocoa, eggnog, milk shakes using straws or tilting head back to make swallowing more comfortable
Avoid discomfort by limiting or eliminating
Tart or acid foods such as citrus juices and fruits
Highly seasoned and spicy foods
Alcohol and cigarettes
Foods that are extreme in temperature

Nausea and vomiting also increase the loss of proteins and water-soluble vitamins necessary for epithelial cell structures. The patient's nurse or a nutritionist should become involved and help to formulate plans for nutritional management [13] (table 7–3; see chapter 8).

Sucrose and refined carbohydrates should be eliminated, as much as possible, from the patient's diet as this will help to reduce the progression of caries and eliminate empty calories. Abrasive foodstuffs such as toast can traumatize the fragile and otherwise compromised mucosa and cause a break in the mucosal barrier to the oral microflora. Citrus fruits and spicy foods can be very irritating to damaged mucosa and should not be given to patients with mucositis or ulcerations.

Xerostomia

Dry mouth, or xerostomia, is a frequent complication of chemotherapy [14] (table 7–4). Some agents in particular, such as Adriamycin, cause dryness of the mucous membranes. Xerostomia is a particularly bothersome problem as it interferes with speech, taste, and eating, and can aggravate an already painful mouth. In addition, adequate salivary flow is important to the remineralization of teeth by maintaining a balance between the loss and replacement of calcium and phosphorous from the surface enamel. Likewise, the balance and number of oral organisms are determined in part by salivary gland output. It has been shown that the bathing of oral mucous membranes with saliva decreases the collection of bacteria in the oropharynx [15].

Xerostomia, therefore, is a significant problem and should not be ignored. Frequent mouth rinses with sterile water or saline, along with other oral hygiene measures, will compensate in part for the lost salivation. Ice water and a straw can be left at bedside for patients to use as needed for dry mouth. A saliva substitute (table 7–5) can be employed

Table 7–4. Common complications of chemotherapy

Problems	Time seen following chemotherapy	Clinical signs and symptoms	Laboratory findings	Treatment	Course
Xerostomia	Variable, Adriamycin predisposes	Dry mouth Thick ropy saliva Diminished taste sensation Metallic taste in mouth Difficulty with speech and nutrition	Noncontributory	Lemon drops (artificial sweeteners) Lemon glycerine swabs Sugarless gum Ice chips Saliva substitute Fluoride (Fl^-) rinses Acidulated Fl^- rinse qd $\times$ 1 min at hs until mucositis Nonacidulated Fl^- rinse as above if acidulated burns	Resolves following treatment
Angular cheilitis	Anytime, but increases with xerostomia Infectious etiology (fungal) in compromised host	Cracking, bleeding, possible exudate and pain in corner of mouth	Smear will demonstrate fungi if *Candida* 5 pp.	Check vertical dimension of teeth Mycolog ointment Vaseline	Watch for secondary infection
Mucositis and ulceration	Direct stomatotoxicity methotrexate: 5–7 days Indirect stomatotoxicity: 10–14 days	Broad shallow to deep ulceration on mucosa Poorly defined borders. May be hemorrhagic. Mucosal erythema. Distinct ovoid deep ulceration with white necrotic centers and dense surrounding band of erythema. May involve keratinized tissue. Often at gingival margin especially in neutropenic patient	Early leukopenia but precedes nadir Neutropenia	Palliation—viscous Xylocaine; Benadryl and Kaopectate; dyclone; or cocaine rinses; benzocaine in orabase for discrete lesions; systemic analgesics; ice chips If secondary infection, parenteral antibiotics to cover gram (−) organisms in addition to conventional flora (gram (+)) Hemorrhage: topical thrombin Soft bland diet as tolerated	Resolves following chemotherapy

Table 7-4 (continued)

Gingival bleeding	Variable, 10–14 days increases with thrombocytopenia	Marginal hemorrhage from gingiva May be spontaneous May be presenting sign	Thrombocytopenia usually not spontaneous if platelets > 15,000/mm³	Platelets Topical thrombin solution soaked in 2×2's Aminocaproic acid Avitene Undisturbed clot D/C mechanical hygiene	Resolves as platelets increase
Mucosal bleeding	10–14 days	Hematoma or bleeding area especially mucosal sites commonly traumatized In case of neutropenic patient, likely chance of secondary infection Beware of sublingual or pharyngeal extension → airway obstruction	Thrombocytopenia Blast crisis with functional decrease in platelets	Remove partial and full dentures. Elimination of orthodontic bands or retainers As above, cover for secondary infection	Resolves with increased platelets Resolving hematoma may extrude granulation plug from healing base; do not disturb
ANUG	Variable: may be unrelated to chemotherapy but incidence increases with neutropenia	Gingival pain and bleeding Fever Lymphadenopathy Gingival necrosis with punched-out papillae Fetor oris	May see leukocytosis if no myelosuppression Fusospirochetal on smear	Parenteral antibiotics, penicillin drug of choice Oral debridement	Resolves following appropriate treatment in 7–10 days
Odontogenic infection in myelosuppressed host	Anytime	Variable, may present with fever of unknown origin, swelling, pain, lymphadenopathy Swelling not consistent finding with neutropenia May be subclinical until increase PMNL	Neutropenia Positive blood culture	Parenteral broad-spectrum antibiotics to cover for opportunistic organisms and normal flora Remove source in presence of adequate cells (WBC > 1,000/mm³ and reasonable PMNL and > 25,000/mm³ platelets)	Variable: depends on organism, counts, location

Table 7–4 (continued

Odontogenic pain of neurotoxic origin	Following neurotoxic agent (for example, vincristine)	Spontaneous, constant, dental pain often mimicking infective pulpitis. Difficult to localize May be bilateral Afebrile No swelling, lymphadenopathy, no significant caries, periodontitis	Pulpal infarct?	Systemic pain medications If pulpal necrosis (localized), may require extraction	Resolves following discontinuation of neurotoxic agent
Salivary gland infection	Anytime, most common in debilitated patient with diminished oral intake and dehydration	Swelling (may be unilateral or bilateral) Pain Suppuration from duct when no myelosuppression Xerostomia Fever	Variable, bacterial cultures → Staph spp. May be viral: cytomegalovirus most common	Antibiotics (parenteral) to cover staph if bacterial Rehydrate Watch for possible airway obstruction	Resolution depends on host status and treatment
Moniliasis	Anytime More likely with prolonged neutropenia, antibiotics, or steroid use	White curds, plaques, ulcerations, tender Affects buccal and palatal mucosa most frequently Corners of mouth may be affected, especially in edentulous patients (see angular cheilitis)	Neutropenia, smear → organisms Positive Ba^{++} swallow with esophageal involvement (watch for false negative)	Prophylactic nystatin swish/swallow, vaginal suppositories if tolerated. Amphotericin if esophageal or systemic involvement suspected Nystatin ointment	Resolves with antifungal treatment or with increased PMNL
Herpes labialis	Anytime	Crops of vesicular lesions that are at or beyond mucocutaneous junction; frequently extraoral with no anatomic distribution	Smear of base of vesicle; increased N/C ratio Viral inclusion bodies	Prevention: keep lubricated; often secondary infection in neutropenic host. Local treatment: neosporin Acyclovir for failure to heal	10–14 days, depending on host resistance

Table 7–5. Formulary of medications for specific oral problems

Antibacterial	
Neosporin (polymyxin B, bacitracin, neomycin)	
Use:	Antibacterial against most commonly occurring bacteria known to be topical invaders
Action:	Antibacterial as above, activity against many bacteria resistant to other antibiotics (for example, *Pseudomonas* and *Staphylococcus*)
Availability:	1- or ½-oz tubes, and foil packet of 1/32 oz
Dose/timing:	Apply to circumoral lesions two to five times daily depending on severity of condition.
Route:	Topical use only
Precautions:	Sensitivity to any of its components; watch for overgrowth of nonsusceptible organisms, including fungi
Manufacturer:	Burroughs Wellcome Co., Research Triangle Park, NC 27709
Acidulated phosphate fluoride (Phos-Flur) (APF)	
Use:	Prevention of dental caries
Action:	Hardening of dental enamel through incorporation into enamel matrix, antibacterial effects
Availability:	250- and 500-ml plastic bottles
Dose/timing:	Children age six and over and all adults rinse vigorously with one or two teaspoonfuls (5 or 10 ml) for one minute and expectorate. Should be done once per day after last meal of the day and following oral hygiene measures
Route:	Oral
Precautions:	Do not swallow; switch to neutral fluoride solution if acidulated fluoride irritates mucosa
Manufacturer:	Hoyt Laboratories, Needham, MA 02194
Neutral sodium fluoride	
Use:	Fluoride uptake lower and more shallow than with acidulated phosphate fluoride; less likely to irritate mucosal lesions
Action:	Same as APF above
Dose:	Same as APF above
Antifungal	
Mycolog (nystatin, neomycin sulfate, gramicidin, triamcinolone acetonide)	
Use:	Angular chelitis where candidal infection is suspected
Actions:	Antiinflammatory, antipruritic, vasoconstrictive, anticandidal, antibacterial
Availability:	Tubes of 15, 30, and 60 g
Dose/timing:	Cream: rub into affected area two to three times daily. Ointment: apply thin film to affected area two to three times daily
Route:	Topical only
Precautions:	Not for use in viral diseases of skin (for example, herpes); hypersensitivity to any component; prolonged use may result in overgrowth of nonsusceptible organisms
Manufacturer:	Squibb & Sons, E.R. Princeton, NJ 08540
Nystatin (Mycostatin oral suspension)	
Use:	Antifungal antibiotic
Action:	Polyene antibiotic that is fungistatic and fungicidal against wide variety of yeasts and yeast-like fungi, binds to yeast and fungi and alters membrane permeability
Availability:	60 ml bottles, 100,000 U per ml; vaginal tablets, 100,000 U
Dose/timing:	1–4 ml (100,000 to 400,000 U) three to four times daily, swish for several minutes if possible and swallow, continue until white count rises and for two days after lesions disappear; hold vaginal suppository in mouth until dissolved
Route:	Oral
Precautions:	Hypersensitivity to any component, solution contains 50% sucrose; may initiate or accelerate dental caries
Manufacturer:	Squibb & Sons, E.R. Princeton, NJ 08540

Ketoconazole

- Use: Oral candidiasis, histoplasmosis
- Action: Antifungal
- Availability: 200 mg tablets
- Dose/timing: 200 mg once per day (400 mg in severe cases)
- Route: Oral
- Precautions: Do not give with antacids
- Manufacturer: Janssen Pharmaceutica, Inc., New Brunswick, NJ 08903

Amphotericin B (Fungizone intravenous)

- Use: Progressive and potentially fatal fungal infections
- Action: Antifungal antibiotic, fungistatic or fungicidal; probably acts by binding to sterols in fungus cell membrane with resultant change in membrane permeability
- Availability: Vials of 50 mg amphotericin B, 41 mg sodium desoxycholate with 25.2 mg sodium phosphate as a buffer
- Dose/timing: Slow intravenous infusion, dosage depends on nature of infection
- Route: IV, not available in United States for oral use
- Precautions: Hypersensitivity, possible life-saving benefit must be balanced against its untoward and dangerous side effects
- Manufacturer: Squibb & Sons, E.R., Princeton, NJ 08540

Bleeding

Thrombin, topical

- Use: Surface bleeding from capillaries and small venules
- Action: Clots fibrinogen directly
- Availability: Package of one 5,000 U.S. (NIH) unit vial of Thrombin, topical and one 5-ml vial isotonic saline with Phemerol as preservative
  Package of 10,000 or 1,000 U.S. (NIH) unit vials
- Dose/timing: Sponge (not wipe) recipient surface and apply 2×2 sponge soaked in topical thrombin to bleeding mucosa and hold with moderate pressure for several minutes. Do not wipe clotted area; repeat as necessary. Sponge may be left in place for extended period of time if necessary. Do not disturb clot that forms with rinsing or manipulation
- Route: Surface bleeding only; do not inject
- Precautions: Sensitivity to any of its components or material of bovine origin. Use solution the day it is prepared; refrigerate if not used for several hours
- Manufacturer: Parke-Davis, Morris Plains, NJ 07950

Microfibrillar collagen hemostat (Avitine)

- Use: Surface mucosal bleeding
- Action: In contact with bleeding surface Avitine attracts platelets that adhere to the fibrils and triggers platelet aggregation. Usually effective in presence of heparinization and in most patients taking aspirin
- Availability: 1- and 5-gm sterile jars in sealed can
- Dose/timing: Compress site with dry sponge immediately prior to applying dry Avitene with smooth dry forceps. Apply pressure over area with dry sponge for one to five minutes depending on severity of bleeding. Can be reapplied if bleeding recurs
- Precautions: Not to be used in closure of mucosal incisions. May potentiate infection; for surface use only. Do not resterilize. Not for injection. Do not moisten with saline or thrombin, should be used dry. Use only enough to produce hemostasis; carefully remove excess material after several minutes
- Manufacturer: Avicon, Inc., Fort Worth, TX 76134

Aminocaproic acid (Amicar)

- Use: Excessive bleeding
- Action: Inhibition of fibrinolysis by inhibition of plasminogen activator substances and antiplasmin activity
- Availability: 20-ml vial with 5.0 gm aminocaproic acid; 25% syrup; 250 mg/ml; tablets—500 mg

Table 7–5 (continued)

Dose/timing:	5 gms orally or intravenously followed by 1- to 1¼-gm doses at hourly intervals
Route:	Intravenous or oral. Benefit from topical use on bleeding mucosa is unknown.
Precautions:	Not for use when there is evidence of active intravascular clotting processes. Use caution in patients with cardiac, hepatic, or renal disease; should be used in situations where benefits outweigh hazards
Manufacturer:	Lederle Laboratories, Pearl River, NY 10965
Gelfoam absorbable gelatin sponge	
Use:	Hemostasis postextraction
Action:	Serves as matrix for clot formation
Availability:	Gelfoam dental packs (size 2 or 4). Each measures 10 × 20 × 7 mm or 20 × 20 × 7 mm respectively, packaged in jars of 15 packs
Precautions:	Question of increased incidence of infection
Manufacturer:	Upjohn Company, Kalamazoo, MI 49001
Pain	
Topical agents	
Viscous Xylocaine (lidocaine HCl)	
Use:	Topical anesthetic for mucous membranes
Action:	Stabilizes neuronal membrane, blocks peripheral nerve conduction
Availability:	2% solution in 100-ml and 450-ml polyethylene squeeze bottles
Dose/timing:	One tablespoonful (15 ml; 300 mg) as needed for pain, not to exceed q3h, or 120 ml in a 24-hr period
Route:	Swish for 30 seconds and expectorate
Precautions:	Increased uptake by traumatized mucosa. Watch for central nervous system (CNS) toxicity
Manufacturer:	Astra Pharmaceutical Products, Worcester, MA 01606
Diphenhydramine hydrochloride (Benadryl)	
Use:	Mixed with Kaopectate 1:1 as topical anesthetic for mucous membranes
Action:	Antihistamine with anticholinergic (drying) and sedative side effects
Availability:	Mixed with kaopectate 1:1 by pharmacy
Dose/timing:	One tablespoonful as needed for pain
Route:	Swish for 30 seconds and expectorate
Precautions:	Concurrent monoamine oxidase inhibitor therapy, narrow angle glaucoma, peptic ulcer, additive effects with other CNS depressants. Watch for excitation or sedation with systemic uptake
Manufacturer:	Upjohn Company, Kalamazoo, MI 49001
Dyclonine hydrochloride (Dyclone)	
Use:	Topical anesthetic for mucous membranes
Action:	Prevents depolarization of nerve fibers
Availability:	0.5% and 1% solutions
Dose/timing:	One tablespoonful as needed for pain
Route:	Swish for 30 seconds and expectorate
Manufacturer:	Dow Pharmaceuticals, Indianapolis, IN 46268
Cocaine	
Use:	Topical anesthetic for mucous membranes
Action:	Anesthesia and vasoconstriction, mucous membrane shrinkage; ? inhibition of uptake of catecholamines by adrenergic nerve terminals
Availability:	Liquid
Dose/timing:	2½–5% applied to mucous membranes. Total dose should be limited
Route:	Swish and expectorate or apply to area
Precautions:	CNS toxicity, euphoria, addiction
Benzocaine (with orabase)	
Use:	Topical anesthetic for localized areas of pain
Action:	Benzocaine held to site by orabase; prevents depolarization of nerve fibers
Availability:	5- and 15-gm tubes
Dose/timing:	Dry mucosa and apply small dab over area as needed for pain
Precautions:	*PDR* warns against use in presence of infection
Manufacturer:	Hoyt Laboratories, Needham, MA 02194

Systemic agents

Acetaminophen

Use:	Mild to moderate pain
Action:	Decreased activity of brain
Availability:	Tablets, capsules
Dose/timing:	300–600 mg every three to four hours
Route:	Oral or rectal
Precautions:	Habituation can occur; hepatic necrosis (large dosages), nephrotoxicity (long-term usage). Potentiates anticoagulant drugs (for example, Coumarin); increases prothrombin time

Codeine sulfate

Use:	Mild to moderate pain
Action:	Narcotic analgesic
Availability:	Tablets or liquid for parenteral use
Dose/timing:	15 mg, 30 mg or 60 mg orally every three to four hours. Maximum analgesic dose is 60 mg
Route:	Oral or parenteral
Precautions:	Drowsiness, nausea, no addiction with short-term use

Meperidine hydrochloride (Demerol)

Use:	Moderate to severe pain
Action:	Narcotic analgesic and sedative. Acts on CNS and organs composed of smooth muscle.
Availability:	Ampules: 25 mg, 50 mg, 75 mg, 100 mg Tablets: 50 mg, 100 mg Syrup: 50 mg per 5 Ml teaspoon
Dose/timing:	50 to 150 mg intramuscularly or orally every three to four hours. IM more effective than oral route.
Precautions:	Hypersensitivity to meperidine; in conjunction with monoamine oxidase inhibitors or CNS or respiratory depressants; chronic obstructive pulmonary disease, hypotension, supraventricular tachycardias, convulsions, severe impairment of hepatic or renal function, hypothyroidism, Addison's disease
Manufacturer:	Winthrop Laboratories, NY, NY 10016

Morphine sulfate

Use:	Moderate to severe pain
Action:	Elevates pain threshold and alters the reaction to painful stimulus
Availability:	Tablets or ampules
Dose/timing:	8–15 mg every three hours
Route:	Oral or parenteral
Precautions:	Respiratory depression, presence of increased intracranial pressure

Hydromorphone hydrochloride (Dilaudid)

Use:	Moderate to severe pain; more potent analgesic than morphine
Action:	Narcotic analgesic, rapid onset; short duration of action
Availability:	Ampules: 1 mg, 2 mg, 3 mg, 4 mg/ml Tablets: 1 mg, 2 mg, 3 mg, 4 mg Rectal suppositories: 3 mg
Dose/timing:	2 mg intramuscularly or subcutaneous every four to six hours 2 mg orally every four to six hours. Up to 3 mg to 4 mg as needed for pain
Route:	Subcutaneous, intramuscular, intravenous, oral, rectal
Precautions:	Respiratory depression, addiction

Sialorrhea

Atropine

Use:	Antisialogog
Action:	Inhibition of smooth muscle and glands innervated by postganglionic cholinergic nerves, CNS excitation or depression depending on dose
Availability:	Vials: 20 ml (0.4 mg/ml) Tablets: 0.4 mg
Dose/timing:	Adults: 0.4–0.6 mg as needed for sialorrhea
Route:	By mouth or intramuscular
Precautions:	Glaucoma, asthma, bradycardia
Manufacturer:	Knoll Pharmaceutical Co., Whippiny, NJ 07981

Table 7–5 (continued)

Xerostomia	
Salivart synthetic saliva	
Use:	Mouth moisturizer, caries inhibition
Action:	Remineralization of surface enamel, replacement of lubricating action of missing saliva
Availability:	50 ml spray cans
Dose/timing:	As needed for xerostomia
Manufacturer:	Westport Pharmaceuticals Inc., Westport, CT 06881
Xerolube	
Use:	Mouth moisturizer, caries inhibition
Action:	Remineralization of surface enamel, replacement of lubricating action of missing saliva, fluoride incorporation into surface enamel
Availability:	As supplied by manufacturer or as prepared by local pharmacy
Dose/timing:	As needed for xerostomia
Manufacturer:	Scherer Laboratories, Inc., Dallas TX 75234

to moisten the mouth and replace the missing constituents of the saliva. Some solutions include fluoride as an added benefit [16]. Salivary stimulation with sugarless lemon candy or glycerine swabs may be helpful if tolerated by the patient. Some patients may prefer sugarless gum but care must be exercised to avoid injury to the compromised mucosa.

An occasional patient will manifest an apparent increase in salivation following chemotherapy. This may result from a change in the viscosity of the saliva or an inability to manage salivary secretions due to dysphagia. An attempt should be made to eliminate all forms of salivary stimulation and reassure the patient that it is a temporary problem. Atropine sulfate (table 7–5) can be used to decrease the salivary flow if not contraindicated due to cardiac considerations.

Pain

The most common oral complaint from patients who have received cancer chemotherapy is pain. The location, severity, and duration of this pain is often atypical and may require special consideration in diagnosis and management [17].

Soft tissue

Pain arising from mucosal tissues is usually a result of chemotherapy-induced direct or indirect stomatotoxicity (table 7–4). Direct stomatotoxicity usually manifests itself within seven days of the onset of chemotherapy and appears to originate from the interruption of mucosal cell division and a resultant thinning out of the mucosa (figures 7–5 and 7–6). Frank ulceration of these thinned areas is the most common oral complication following chemotherapy [14, 18]. Submucosal changes occur as well and may contribute to the discomfort experienced from mucosal toxicity [19]. Tissues may appear erythematous, glistening, and swollen as well as be sensitive to any manipulation. There may be constant, spontaneous pain that limits speech, sleep, and nutrition. Patient's severity of pain can vary, ranging from mild soreness in an isolated area to extreme and diffuse pain requiring narcotics for control. Indirect stomatotoxicity manifests itself greater than seven days from the initiation of chemotherapy. The incidence and severity of this phenomenon are often directly related to the degree of preexisting mucosal disease and the degree and duration of marrow suppression.

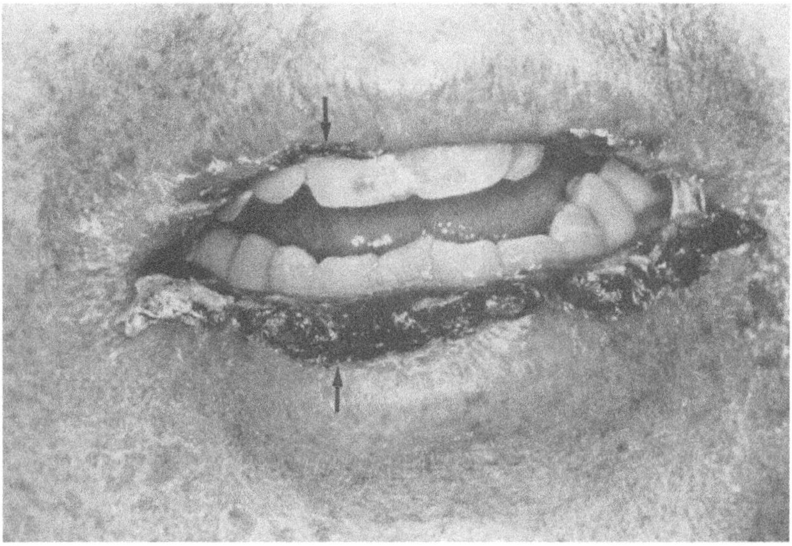

Figure 7–5. 38-year-old female treated with 5-FU for colon carcinoma. Note severe labial mucosa breakdown that extends to the mucocutaneous junction *(arrows)*. All oral mucosal tissues sloughed within several days of chemotherapy.

The pain from both direct and indirect stomatoxicity is managed medically with palliation until the mucosa heals. Pain from isolated areas of mucositis or ulceration on the tongue, buccal mucosa, or gingiva may be best managed with topical anesthetic ointments (for example, benzocaine in Orabase) (table 7–5) applied to dry mucosa as often as needed. Orabase serves to hold the benzocaine in place for longer periods of time. Such ointments avoid the unpleasantness of total mucosal anesthesia that results from anesthetic rinses. When the pain originates from several broad areas of mucosa or sites inaccessible to benzocaine ointment, topical anesthetic rinses such as Viscous Xylocaine, Dyclone, Kaopectate in Benadryl, or even 2½ to 5% cocaine rinses must be employed (table 7–5). Milk of Magnesia, often mixed with Benadryl, should be avoided as it has a significant drying affect on the mucosa. Anesthetic rinses have the disadvantages of unpleasant taste, short periods of activity, and varying toxicities from mucosal uptake which limits the frequency of use. Topical anesthetics have a variable effect as some patients may have pain relief that lasts for an hour or more and others claim no benefit at all. Several agents should be tried until one is found that is tolerated and of some benefit. In situations where topical anesthetic rinses are not tolerated, or are ineffective, consideration must be given to systemic analgesics or narcotics for pain control. Acetaminophen, codeine, meperidine hydrochloride, morphine or hydromorphone hydrochloride, depending on pain severity and the individual pain threshold, will usually allow the patient enough relief for sleep and consumption of at least bland liquids (table 7–5). Aspirin-containing drugs must never be given to these patients because of ill effects on platelet function. Mucosal pain secondary to mucositis is

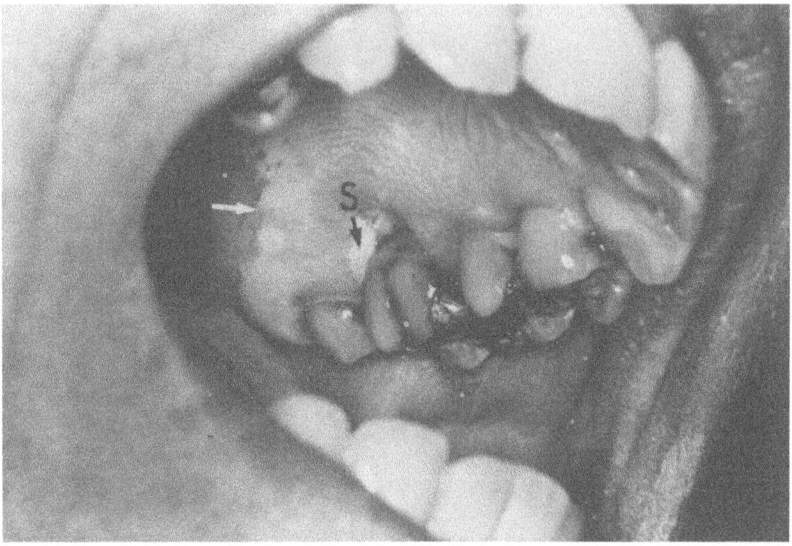

Figure 7–6. 38-year-old woman with acute promyelocytic leukemia at her nadir from chemotherapy (WBC = 660/mm^3, neutrophils = 0%). Note sloughing of palatal mucosa that extends to junction of hard and soft palate *(arrow)*. Note also sloughing *(S)* of gingival tissue on palatal surface of maxillary left first molar. Patient was febrile and mildly symptomatic in this area during her nadir but became septic with a return of neutrophils to her peripheral blood. Exudate appeared around the tooth and pain necessitated its removal, which resolved all signs and symptoms of infection.

a common sequela of cancer treatment, is frustrating to the clinician, and has been used by patients as a reason for refusing additional chemotherapy.

Odontogenic

The presentation of odontogenic infections is clearly altered in immunosuppressed patients (table 7–4). A rise in temperature may be the only indication of infection as the lack of inflammatory response may eliminate or decrease pain as a presenting symptom. Sensitivity to palpation, percussion, and chewing may be absent. When pain from a periapical or periodontal site is present, however, it is managed in the usual way with systemic analgesics or narcotics. The selection of specific agents and the route of delivery may be altered by the patient's propensity for bleeding and infection, the risk of respiratory depression, and the masking of cerebral signs of impairment.

Neurotoxicity

Some chemotherapeutic agents, such as vincristine (Oncovin), are neurotoxic [20]. Patients may complain of constant, severe, deep, often bilateral mandibular pain that is pulpal in nature but has no identifiable odontogenic or mucosal source. The absence of mucosal alterations, caries, periodontal disease, or typical radiographic signs of infection, and the bilateral presentation point to neurotoxicity. Patients should be given adequate systemic narcotics as indicated and reassured that the pain will resolve with the discontinuation of the offending chemotherapeutic drug.

Other sources

Pulpal infiltration by leukemic cells has also been proposed as a cause of dental pain in the absence of dental disease [21]. The incidence of this phenomenon is unknown but it should be kept in mind in order to avoid needless extraction of teeth.

Temporomandibular joint pain, or acute myofacial pain dysfunction syndrome, is not uncommon in the population at large. One might expect to see an increased incidence of stress-related temporomandibular joint pain in cancer patients due to their diagnosis and treatment. Such does not seem to be the case, however, but careful history taking and examination of patients with facial pain for trismus, pain, and/or deviation on wide jaw opening or tenderness of one of the muscles of mastication may reveal a self-limiting problem that excludes infection as a cause of facial pain [22].

Bleeding

The oral cavity is often the first site to manifest coagulopathies in the otherwise healthy patient and may herald the finding of malignancy in an undiagnosed patient [7,10]. As stated previously, chemotherapy predisposes to oral bleeding in two ways. The gingival crevice, because of preexisting ulceration from periodontal disease, is prone to either spontaneous or traumatic bleeding. The compromised mucosa, combined with the indirect effect of marrow suppression and resultant thrombocytopenia as well as the disease itself and treatment-induced coagulapathies, lead to a high incidence of oral bleeding problems (table 7–4).

Oral bleeding secondary to thrombocytopenia can manifest in a variety of ways. For example, petechiae may often be observed on the lips, soft palate, or floor of mouth. Submucosal hematomas may also be found in the just-mentioned locations as well as the buccal mucosa and lateral borders of the tongue along the occlusal plane. Trauma from the teeth can lead to hematoma formation followed several days later by mucosal breakdown over the hematoma. Eventually an extrusion of a broad-based exophytic plug of granulation tissue may develop. These plugs of tissue should not be removed while the mucosa heals underneath from the periphery, as they will slough within a few days. Larger hematomas are less common but are a concern for two reasons. First, they may extend posteriorly to involve the tongue or pharyngeal wall and compromise the airway. Second, these collections of blood are potential niduses for infection (figure 7–7). Bleeding from the gingiva is the most common source for oral hemorrhage and can become a particularly difficult problem to manage. The gingival crevice, often ulcerated before chemotherapy, becomes more prone to bleeding with time. Levels of plaque and calculus increase around the teeth, and minimal trauma produces oozing in the presence of thrombocytopenia (figure 7–3). Spontaneous gingival oozing may occur in some patients with greater than 50,000 platelets/mm^3 or may not occur with less than 1,000 platelets/mm^3 (figure 7–2). In addition to platelet number, qualitative platelet activity, capillary fragility, and other coagulopathies all combine to predispose to oral bleeding.

Patients with acute myelogenous leukemia may have gingival hypertrophy secondary

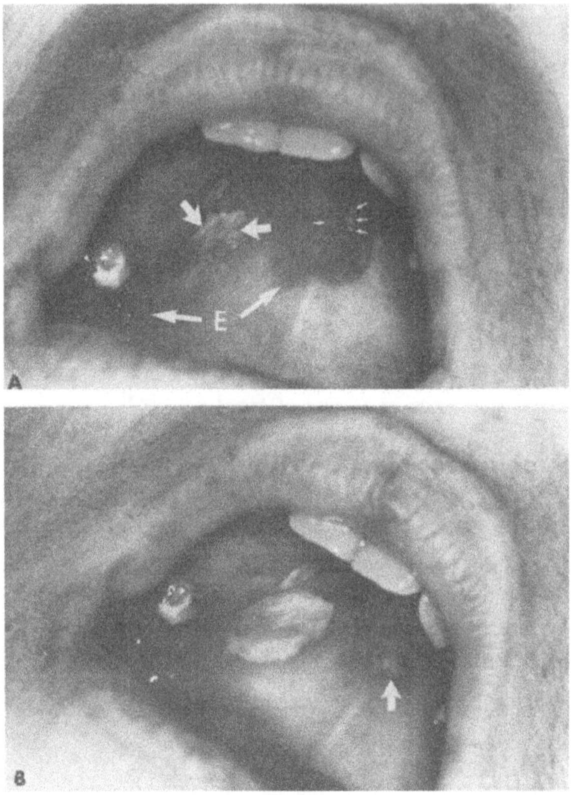

Figure 7–7.

A. 36-year-old woman with acute myelogenous leukemia seen for fever of unknown origin (WBC = $300/mm^3$, neutrophils = 0%, platelets = $30{,}000/mm^3$). Note extensive area of ecchymosis *(E)*, large deeply infected palatal ulceration *(large arrows)*, and several small ulcerated areas *(small arrows)*.

B. Same patient as above, 3 days later (WBC = $400/mm^3$; neutrophils = 2% [first appearance of neutrophils for 11 days]). Note that the several ulcerated areas on palate have coalesced to one large infected ulceration *(arrow)*.

C. Same patient as above, six days later (WBC = $6{,}000/mm^3$; neutrophils = 44% [up from WBC = $1{,}700/mm^3$ and neutrophils = 28% the previous day]). Note that the large ulceration *(arrow)* appears clean and that the infection has largely resolved with the return of neutrophils to the peripheral blood.

to leukemic infiltrates. As bleeding is more of a problem in this setting, radiotherapy may be necessary to reduce the tumor infiltrate.

Spontaneous gingival bleeding must be managed carefully as it can persist with the thrombocytopenia, cause loss of clotting factors and whole blood, and be particularly upsetting to the patient, visitors, and those caring for the patient. Management consists of stopping all oral hygiene measures including rinsing. Large clots should be debrided and 2×2 sponges soaked in topical thrombin applied to the area and held in place until no longer needed (table 7–5). It may be possible to remove the sponge after several minutes;

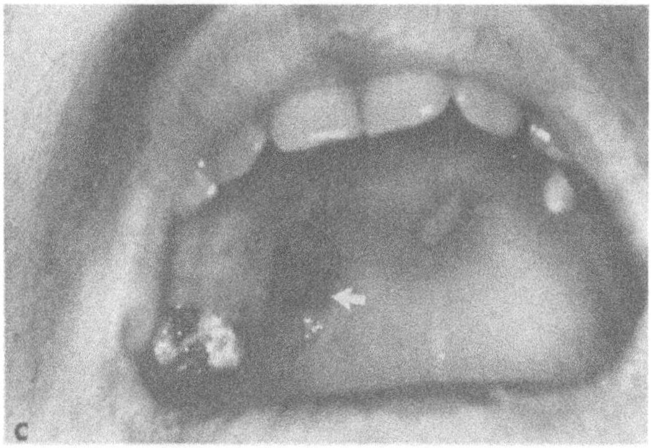

if bleeding begins again a new sponge should be held in place with pressure for a longer period of time. Topical thrombin is usually quite effective, but the clots formed are fragile and easily disrupted. In a situation where topical thrombin and pressure fails to stop the bleeding, aminocaproic acid (EACA; Amicar) has been utilized in the same manner with some success (table 7–5). However, most authorities advise against the use of Amicar in the presence of renal impairment or disseminated intravascular coagulation, both not uncommon in this patient population. Microfibrillar collagen (Avitine) has been used for superficial abrasions or ulcerations that result in mucosal oozing but has little benefit over topical thrombin for hemostasis (table 7–5). The use of platelet transfusions is dependent on the threat of bleeding into the brain, gastrointestinal tract, or other vital organ. Antiplatelet antibodies arise from the overuse of platelet transfusions and their use for oral bleeding must therefore be weighed carefully. Again, patients and those caring for them must be cautioned against any manipulation of the gingival tissues such as chewing, brushing, or even rinsing that can prolong the bleeding indefinitely.

Infection

The majority of cancer patients who die following chemotherapy succumb to infections. Since the oral cavity is a reservoir of pathogenic organisms, any oral infection must be closely monitored in these patients (see chapter 3 and 4).

Chelitis

Because of the dehydrating and xerostomic effects from some chemotherapeutic agents, angular chelitis and generalized lip cracking are common findings in these patients (table 7–4) (figure 7–8). Aside from the discomfort that patients have with painful, dry lips, there is the very real potential that these fissures may become secondarily infected with one or more of a variety of pathogenic organisms, especially *Candida spp.* Such infections are difficult to treat, often spread well beyond the lips, and interfere with movement of the labial musculature and mucosa. Mycolog cream can be applied to suspected areas of candida infection at the corners of the mouth (table 7–5). Vaseline can be employed as often as necessary to keep the lips from drying out.

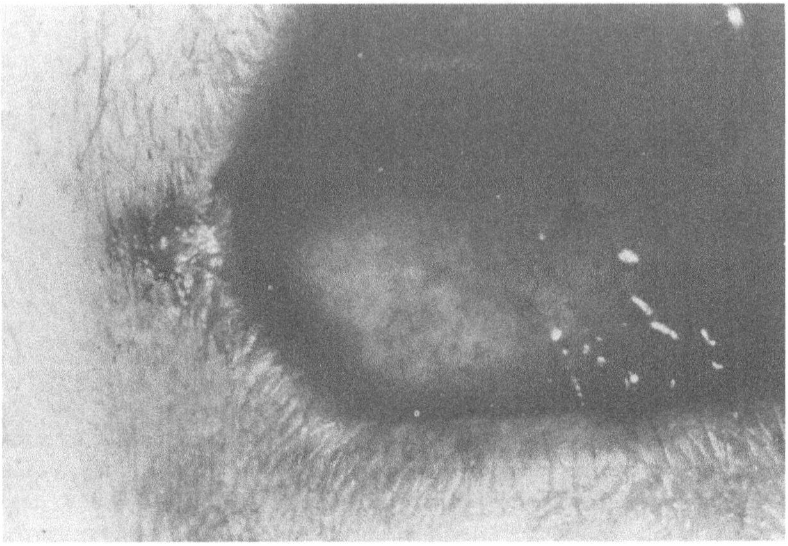

Figure 7–8. 67-year-old woman with Adriamycin-induced xerostomia. Note cracking and erythema at commissure of mouth. Cultures were positive for *Candida spp.*

Bacterial

Mixed bacterial infections of the oral cavity are relatively common in these patients. With the neutropenia-induced shift in the oral flora from gram (+) to gram (−) and anaerobic organisms, chemotherapy and the disease itself [23], the mouth serves as a warm, dark, moist culture medium for growth of these organisms. Recent studies have demonstrated the high incidence of mixed as well as pure gram (−) anaerobes from otherwise healthy patients with dental abscesses [24].

Soft tissue infection usually begins as an ulcerated area that becomes infected with one or more of the following organisms: *Pseudomonas spp., Serratia spp., Klebsiella spp., Escherichia coli* and *Candida albicans* [25]. Gram (−) bacillary infections, except for *Pseudomonas,* usually appear as a gray or creamy white exudate on an ulcerated base with or without a surrounding band of erythema. This area may enlarge over a short period of time and may deepen such that rolled borders occur around a central depressed area (figure 7–9). This is often seen on the tongue but can occur anywhere in the mouth. The amount of pain is variable and is often less than would be expected from the appearance of the lesion. In the profoundly neutropenic patient, the physical findings of swelling, local heat, exudate, or fluctuance and regional adenopathy may be absent. Localized erythema and pain may be present, however, and in the presence of fever should be treated as a potentially serious infection until proven otherwise [26].

Soft tissue infection also commonly occurs around the cervices of teeth where ulceration and necrosis are common pretreatment findings. Acute gingival infection can occur suddenly and may take on the appearance of acute necrotizing ulcerative gingivitis (ANUG),

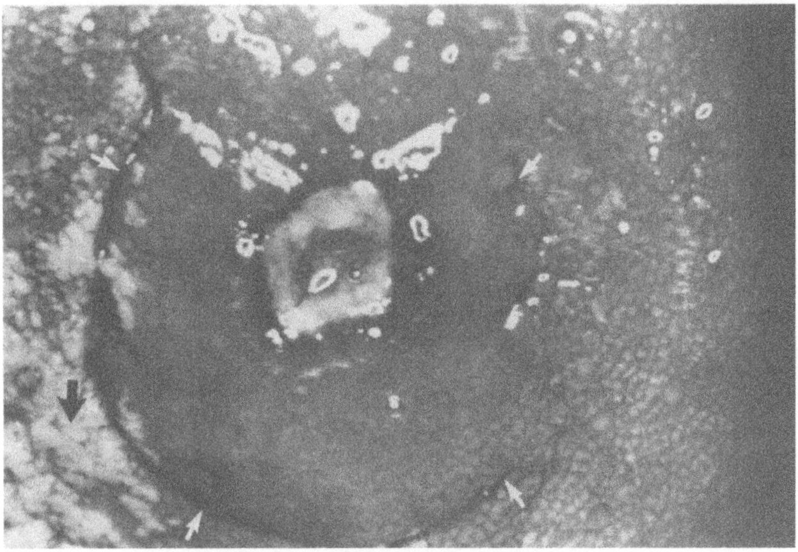

Figure 7–9. 54-year-old neutropenic patient with tongue ulcer of three weeks' duration. Note close-up view of 1×1 cm ulceration surrounded by donut-shaped swelling *(arrows)*. White material *(arrow)* is nystatin-stained debris. Infection resolved with Metronidazole.

without the usual band of erythema. ANUG is a fusospirochetal infection usually seen in young adults who are stressed, fatigued, and who have poor nutritional intake and oral hygiene (table 7–4). Cancer patients would appear to be particularly susceptible to this infection. ANUG is usually accompanied by fever, lymphadenopathy, and pain which is often severe. These areas of papillary necrosis can spread from the interdental areas to involve more of the attached gingiva around the teeth as well as large areas of the palate. The degree and duration of neutropenia particularly predispose to this type of infection. Soft tissue infection (figure 7–10) of any size should be monitored closely as systemic involvement can quickly develop.

Treatment of these soft tissue infections depends on several factors. No single antibiotic agent is effective against all potential causative oral organisms; multiple drug combinations given parenterally are usually necessary to cover for systemic spread of infection, especially in the neutropenic patient. Difficulty often arises in determining which mucosal lesions represent a threat to the patient. It may be difficult to differentiate among soft tissue sloughing (from direct or indirect stomatoxicity), *Candida* that may not have its characteristic appearance, superficial infection that may be walled off from the systemic circulation, or deep invasive infection that requires immediate attention. Often the decision to institute antibiotics must rely on fewer hard signs or symptoms of infection such as fluctuance, swelling, and significant pain, and more on the basis of fever, localized discomfort, or clinical evidence of sepsis. The potential seriousness of these oral lesions lends to the use of antibiotics sooner than would be contemplated in the immunocompetent host. Experi-

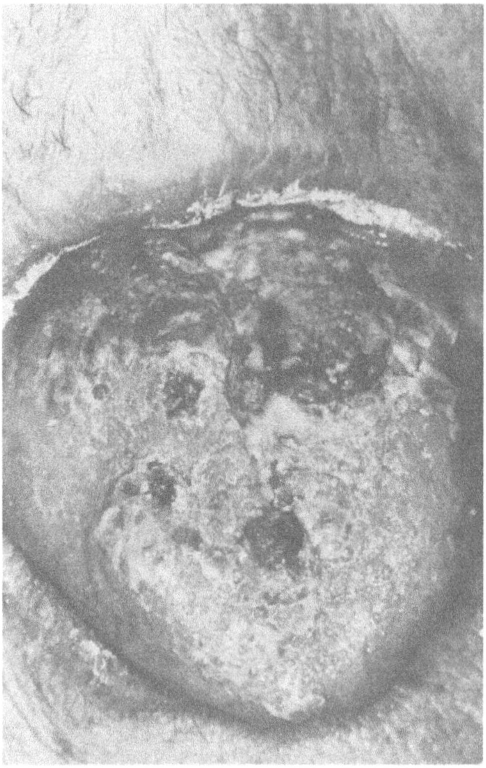

Figure 7–10. 67-year-old female with four-year history of chronic myelogenous leukemia, recently treated with chemotherapy for blast crisis (WBC = $570/mm^3$, neutrophils = 81%). Patient was febrile and had significant tongue pain and dysphagia. No other sites of infection were found, and patient died of sepsis four days later. Tongue cultures grew out multiple gram negative organisms.

ence must be gained in differentiating between these different lesions, as needless use of antibiotics is to be discouraged and nonbacterial infections should be managed with other more specific agents.

Soft tissue lesions should be kept clean to decrease both the amount of growth media for organisms and the discomfort to the patient. This should be done carefully with wet 2×2 sponges, Q-tips, sterile saline, or water and suction. Care must be exercised as overzealous debridement may cause bacteremias, the incidence, nature, and sequelae of which are still poorly understood.

A swab for aerobic and anaerobic cultures may be helpful in identifying a specific organism or organisms. However, many are mixed infections and in the neutropenic patient must be managed with multiple-drug parenteral antibiotics. Patients should be started on broad-spectrum antibiotics until culture results are available. All cultured organisms should be noted and care exercised before assuming that any organism is a contaminant. Infections from obscure organisms have been documented in these patients and the oral cavity can serve as a source of a large number of unusual pathogens [27].

A biopsy of the area in question is usually of little but academic interest and may pose a significant threat as patients are usually pancytopenic when these lesions occur. History, laboratory values, and appearance to the trained eye will usually disclose the nature of the lesions, and this determines the appropriate management.

Odontogenic, or periapical, infections should be managed nonsurgically if possible until the patient's counts return to near normal (see table 7–4). Dental infections may remain quiescent during profound neutropenia until the patient gets a return of an adequate number of neutrophils to the peripheral blood. Neutrophils marginate to the site of infection, pus is formed and the patient may become symptomatic (see figure 7–6). Medical management of localized infection as long as possible while the white count returns to near normal may be controversial, but ensures that an extraction-associated bacteremia will not cause an overwhelming sepsis.

If the patient is already at his or her WBC nadir or is expected to be within several days, invasive procedures such as extractions or endodontics will likely be contraindicated (see chapter 5). The bacteremia associated with these procedures could seed a distant site with pathogenic organisms that have been localized by the patient's host defenses. Extraction sites require several days or longer to reepithelialize because of the decreased cell renewal time of mucosa subjected to chemotherapy. Root canals require weeks or months for definitive evaluation of success or failure, and such time usually does not exist. Venting the pulp chamber, however, is preferable to an extraction in a situation where bleeding is a concern, where surgical drainage is possible by pulpectomy, and as a temporary solution to pulpitis until an extraction can be accomplished safely. Standard endodontic principles such as rubber dams and sterile instruments are employed. Care must be exercised to avoid perforating the root apex and introducing organisms into the systemic circulation [28]. Extractions are preferable, however, in situations where the infection is localized to an identifiable tooth and is not controlled by antibiotics and nonsurgical therapy. In rare situations an extraction may be deemed less threatening to the patient than any other alternative, and this should be performed as atraumatically as possible with appropriate broad-spectrum, parenteral antibiotic coverage. Sharp alveolar bone should be smoothed and an attempt made at primary closure to promote healing as the need for drainage is unlikely in the presence of neutropenia.

Extractions may become necessary with platelet counts under 20,000/mm^3. In situations where thrombocytopenia is the major concern, a platelet transfusion just prior to the procedure may raise the number of circulating platelets to a more acceptable level. Gelfoam in the socket with primary closure over the wound will usually suffice for hemostasis (see table 7–5). The use of gelfoam raises the concern of introducing a foreign body as a nidus for bacterial growth. Our group has used gelfoam in over 200 extraction sites without subsequent infection, but all were done in the presence of antibiotic coverage. The need for hemostasis should be weighed against the threat of infection, however, as disruption of the primary clot may lead to prolonged bleeding in the face of thrombocytopenia. Large hematomas may extravasate around the surgical area but are usually self-limiting. They require frequent examinations, however, to check for extention under the tongue or toward the pharyngeal wall.

An occasional patient will manifest a spontaneous, essentially asymptomatic, facial swelling in the presence of pancytopenia. In a series of such patients it was found that all had some degree of maxillofacial mucosal infection or inflammation [29]. Some patients had diffuse mucosal ulceration while others had severe but localized gingival breakdown. Pericoronitis and maxillary sinus infection were also implicated as possible causes. In some cases the swelling heralded the return of polymorphonuclear leukocytes to the peripheral blood and appeared to be caused by a pooling of edema that formed near the involved mucosal surfaces. In other cases, however, the patient was at his/her nadir and the swelling resolved spontaneously at least several days prior to any sign of marrow regeneration. The evidence from this small series points to a nonspecific swelling that may represent an ineffectual response to bacterial toxins in the area. Because of the patient's counts it is considered of little benefit to attempt aspiration of these areas. If concern exists that the swelling represents a collection of neutrophils or pus, and the patient's WBC and neutrophil counts support the possibility, surgical drainage should be carried out. If, however, the patient is severely neutropenic and afebrile, the facial swelling can be observed for 24 to 48 hours with prophylactic intravenous antibiotics if deemed necessary. Attempts to manage oral infections in immunosuppressed patients with oral antibiotics often fails and necessitates a change to parenteral broad-spectrum coverage for a deteriorating situation.

The difficulty, then, is knowing when to carry out invasive procedures (for example, biopsy, aspiration, scalings, or extractions), and when to wait and manage the problem medically until the patient can respond immunologically to the inevitable bacteremia that results from such procedures. With proper antibiotic management, patients with oral infection rarely succumb to these infections; given this, they should not be challenged by procedures that antibiotics and platelets alone cannot handle.

Fungal

Fungal infections, usually *Candida spp.,* are also common in this patient population [30, 31]. The usual predisposing factors that increase the risk of fungal infection include steroids and antibiotics, denture use, debilitation, a history of diabetes, along with the degree and duration of neutropenia. The ultimate concern is extention of fungal organisms to the esophagus or bronchus that can result in a serious if not fatal infection. Oral candidiasis can be difficult to differentiate clinically from sloughing mucosal tissue and some gram negative infections. Wet mount preparations in 10% KOH that demonstrate pseudohyphae when taken from a clinically suspicious area are diagnostic (see table 7–4). Since *Candida spp.* are a normal inhabitant in the mouths of 25 to 60% of the general population [32,33], cultures for *Candida* are of dubious value.

Intraoral candidal lesions may appear as superficial, raised, white punctate crops or patches with or without an erythematous margin (figures 7–11, 7–12). Removal of the patch with a tongue blade leaves an ulcerated base that may be hemorrhagic. Patients may be started on nystatin swish and swallow at the initiation of chemotherapy, but

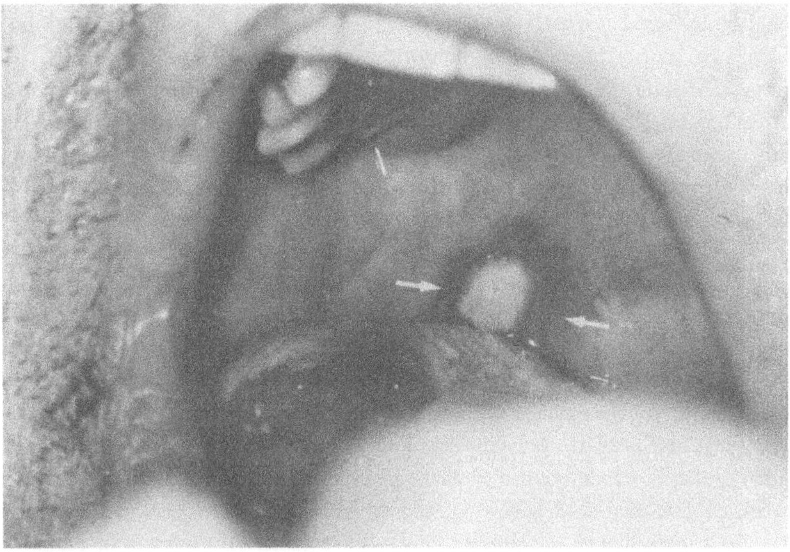

Figure 7–11. 56-year-old male with acute myelogenous leukemia. Patient was at his nadir from Ara C chemotherapy and had multiple areas of intraoral *Candida*-like lesions. Note patch of thick, raised creamy white area with a significant band of erythema *(arrows)*. Cultures for fungi were negative in spite of clinical picture of *Candida*.

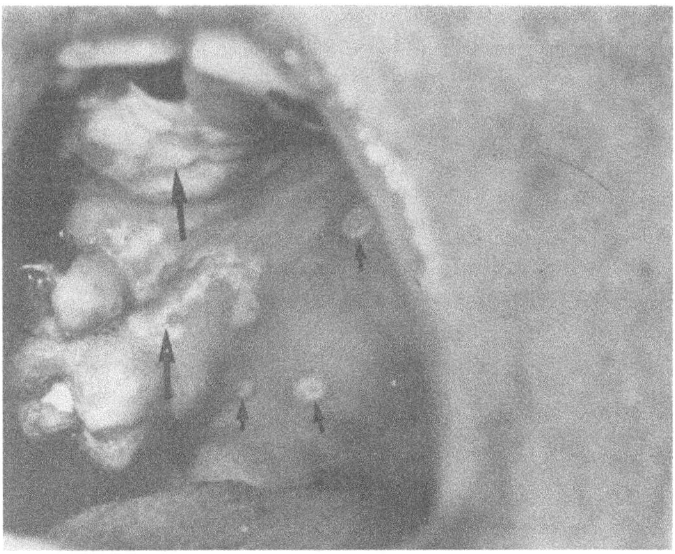

Figure 7–12. 48-year-old woman with acute myelogenous leukemia in relapse. Note crop of small ulcers *(small arrows)* that have coalesced into larger areas of candidiasis *(large arrows)*.

when oral signs of *Candida* appear, the dosage and frequency of the nystatin rinses should be increased (see table 7–5). The addition of nystatin vaginal suppositories will prolong the contact of the medication with the fungus and may improve the overall therapy. The ability of antifungal agents to prevent the onset of candidiasis is controversial [2,32,34,35]. The rationale is that they may prolong the onset of oral candidiasis to a time when the patient's peripheral white count is returning. It is recommended, therefore, that patients expected to become neutropenic from chemotherapy be started on at least thrice daily rinses with 100,000 or more units of nystatin. This should be continued until the neutrophil count begins to rise following the nadir. At least two to three minutes of swishing is desirable, (longer if tolerated), followed by swallowing the medication. Some patients will have problems with nausea and thus be prevented from swallowing, if not swishing, the solution. It should be kept in mind that Mycostatin contains 50% sucrose. Ketoconazole is another antifungal agent that is marketed in pill form and taken once per day (see table 7–5). Gentian violet is a traditional standard in antifungal therapy that may be particularly effective in Nystatin-resistant cases. The disadvantages of gentian violet, however, are that it stains the mucosa purple, obscures the appearance of any lesions that may need following, and on occasion causes superficial tissue necrosis [36]. The patient should be followed closely for evidence of extension of the infection to the esophagus or lungs. Any signs or symptoms suggestive of candidal esophagitis should be evaluated with a barium swallow, and consideration given to prompt intervention with systemic antifungal agents such as amphotericin B (see table 7–5.) False negative esophograms can occur, however, in the presence of complete esophageal mucosal denudation [37] (figure 7–13).

The return of polymorphonuclear leukocytes to the peripheral circulation usually resolves the fungal infection rapidly, and in some patients marrow regeneration may be heralded by a spontaneous sloughing of the oral candidal plaques about 24 hours prior to the appearance of neutrophils on a peripheral smear [38] (see figure 7–7).

Viral

The most common virus affecting the lower face and mouth of these patients is herpes labialis (see table 7–4). Leukemic patients may have very low interferon titers and impaired delayed hypersensitivity and are therefore more susceptible to disseminated forms of herpes infections [2]. Intraoral herpes, rare in the immunocompetent host, may be mistaken for other phenomenon or infections, as the lesions may become secondarily infected with a fungus or bacteria. Viral lesions within the mouth do not usually demonstrate a blister appearance but quickly coalesce and appear as bacterial infections. Intraoral viral infection typically begins as a small cluster of round ulcers that spread and later coalesce to form more irregular ulcerations. The lesions may have a central, usually gray or off-white, area of necrosis and a surrounding band of erythema, depending on marrow status. A culture may be helpful in determining which intraoral lesions are of viral etiology. A smear of the base of the vesicle may show an increase in the nuclear/cytoplasmic ratio and viral inclusion bodies. Extraoral herpes usually begins at or near the vermillion border; unlike typical labialis in the immunocompetent patient, however, the lesions can multiply and spread beyond the vermillion border to involve larger areas of the face (figure 7–14.). Since

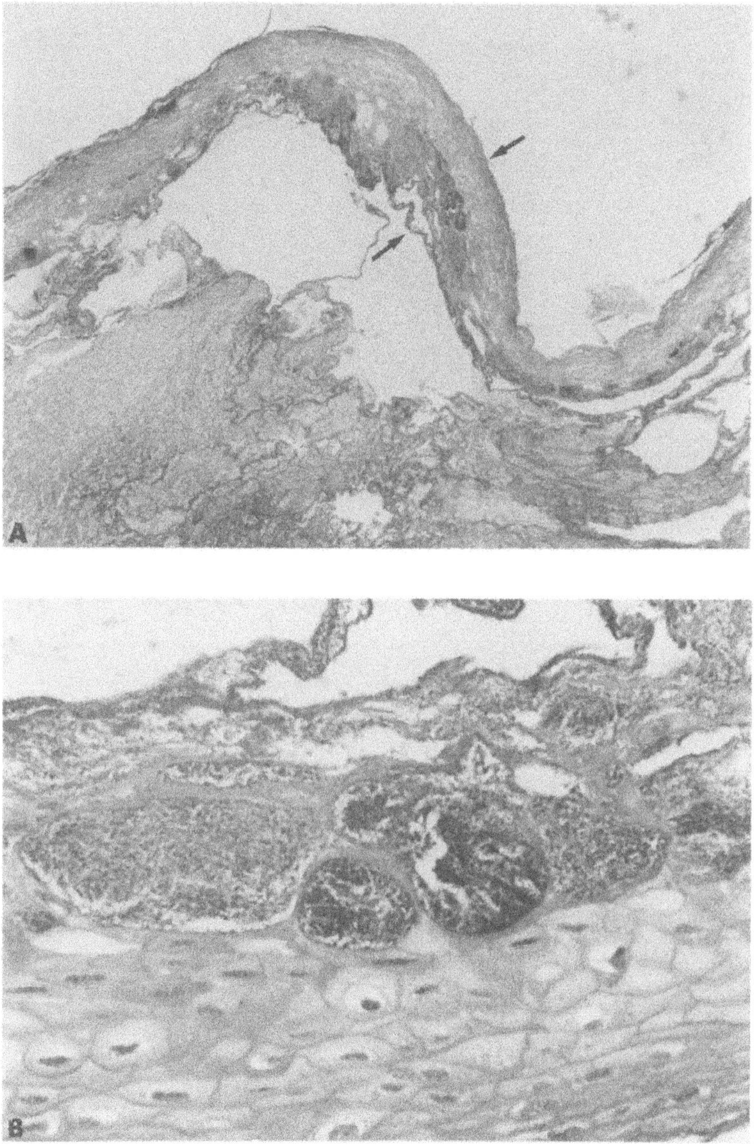

Figure 7–13.

A. 33-year-old female with acute myelogenous leukemia and six days out from induction chemotherapy (WBC = 90/mm^3, neutrophils = 0%). Note autopsy specimen from esophagus which demonstrates atrophy, necrosis, and sloughing of epithelium. Patient had negative barium swallow 24 hours prior to death due to fungal sepsis.

B. High-power view of area in figure 7–13 **A** *(arrows).* Note mucosal atrophy and large collection of bacteria and fungus that have invaded tissue.

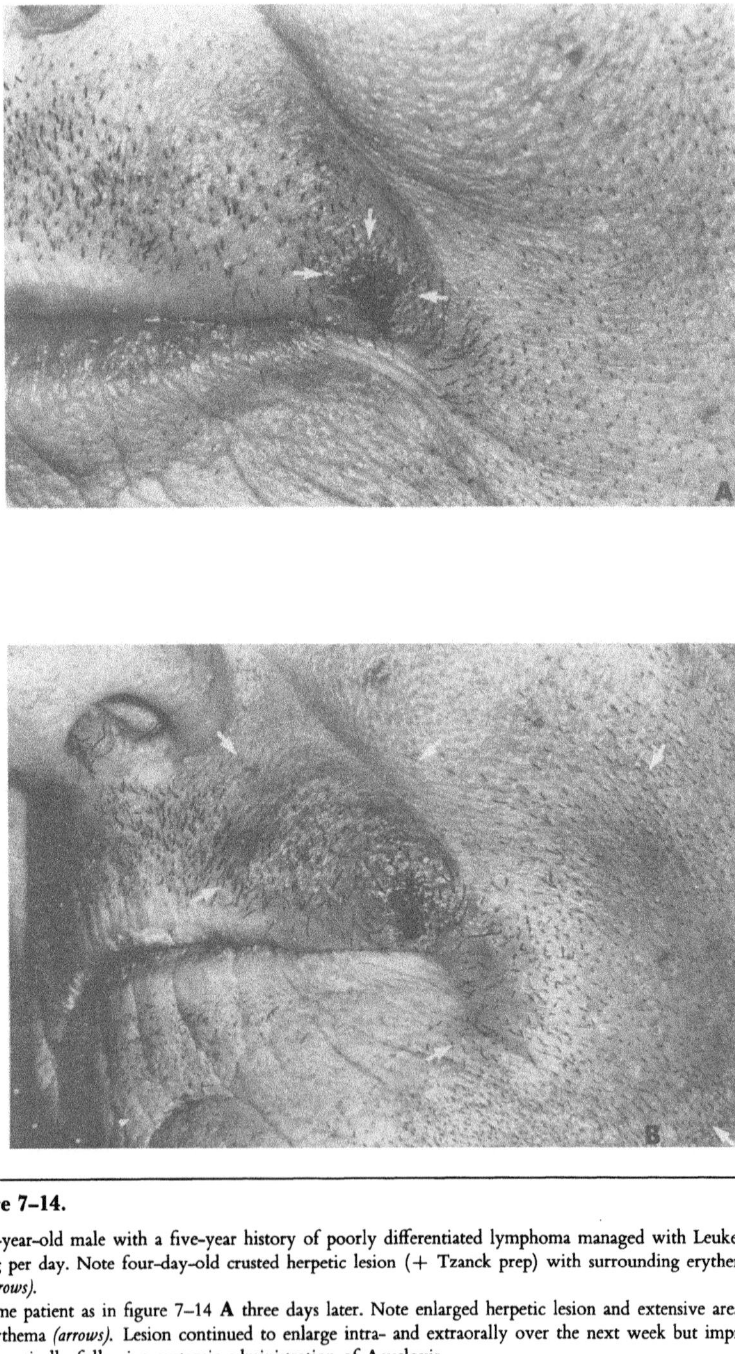

Figure 7–14.

A. 61-year-old male with a five-year history of poorly differentiated lymphoma managed with Leukeran 2 mg per day. Note four-day-old crusted herpetic lesion (+ Tzanck prep) with surrounding erythema *(arrows)*.

B. Same patient as in figure 7–14 **A** three days later. Note enlarged herpetic lesion and extensive area of erythema *(arrows)*. Lesion continued to enlarge intra- and extraorally over the next week but improved dramatically following systemic administration of Acyclovir.

lip cracking is common with these lesions, the lips should be covered with an ointment (for example, Vaseline or Neosporin) to prevent cracking and reduce the possibility of secondary infection (see table 7–5). Various anti-herpes ointments are available that can be applied as needed for dryness and may be helpful in reducing the severity, longevity and potential for secondary infection. Severely neutropenic patients may experience prolonged and extensive herpetic lesions that can result in significant morbidity. Intra- or extra-oral herpes that does not resolve in the usual time period will likely respond to newer agents such as Acyclovir [39,40].

SUMMARY

Both the increasing number of patients receiving cancer chemotherapy and the intensity of the drug regimens employed have resulted in a larger number of patients who need careful evaluation and management of a variety of unusual oral problems. From the preceding discussion it is clear that a thorough oral examination is of considerable importance in the overall prechemotherapy evaluation of the patient. Existing and potential oral disease can be identified from a thorough patient history and examination. This information, along with a consideration for the patient's disease, prognosis and laboratory values, allows for realistic planning for dental management prior to, during, and following the cancer chemotherapy. Preventive measures for eradication and control of oral disease are never more important than with this patient group. The early establishment of a good working relationship with the patient and those caring for him/her, and an understanding of the importance of compliance in oral hygiene measures will eliminate needless chemotherapy-induced morbidity and mortality.

Of all the oral problems encountered by these patients, pain, bleeding, and infection are the most troublesome and difficult to manage. Both direct and indirect stomatotoxicity often result in significant and prolonged oral pain, and its management is too often only palliative. In fact, direct stomatotoxicity in the form of painful mucositis is a dose-limiting factor for some chemotherapy protocols. Mucosal pain will ultimately be brought under better control in the future with both prevention of direct stomatotoxicity and longer-acting topical anesthetics. Oral bleeding, although troublesome, is rarely life-threatening. Its occurrence in the mouth, however, interferes with hygiene, speech, and adequate nutrition. Gingival bleeding is often a function of periodontal health and therefore is largely preventable. Infection, the major cause of death in these patients, presents the greatest challenges in dental management. The mouth, which contains the largest number and variety of pathogenic organisms in immunocompetent patients, becomes a major potential source of local or systemic infection in the immunosuppressed cancer patient. The availability of the newer broad-spectrum parenteral antibiotics allows for control of most oral organisms, but problems of causative species identification and development of resistant strains often renders antibiotic management of the oral flora empiric at best.

The increasing number of published articles on oral complications of cancer chemotherapy indicates a greater awareness of the importance of the mouth in the overall management of patients on chemotherapy. The interest in these problems will ultimately lead to improvements in prevention and management and allow for more aggressive chemotherapy that will increase survival rates and improve the quality of life for these patients.

REFERENCES

1. Lockhart PB, Sonis ST: Utilization of inpatient dental consultation services. Spec Care Dent 1:18–21, 1981.
2. Madhavan T, Van Slyck EJ: Infections in acute leukemia. Drug Ther 7:49–58, 1977.
3. Hupp JR, Booth DF, Kilfore TB: Alternatives to dental extractions in leukemia. N Engl J Med 295:676–677, 1976.
4. Schiliro G, et al.: Dental care in leukemia. N Engl J Med 296:109, 1977.
5. Ostchega Y: Preventing and treating cancer chemotherapy's oral complications. Nursing 10:47–52, 1980.
6. Stafford R, Sonis ST, Lockhart P, Sonis A: Oral pathoses as diagnostic indicators in leukemia. Oral Surg 50:134–139, 1980.
7. Stafford R, Lockhart P, Sonis A, Sonis S: Hematologic parameters of oral involvement in the presentation of acute leukemia. J Oral Med (in press).
8. Sconyers JR, Crawford JJ, Moriarity JD: Relationship of bacteremia to toothbrushing in patients with periodontitis. Am Dent Assoc 87:616–622, 1973.
9. Drapkin MS: Endocarditis after the use of an oral irrigation device. *Ann Intern Med* 87:455, 1977.
10. Lynch MA, Ship II: Initial oral manifestation of leukemia. J Am Dent Assoc 75:932–940, 1967.
11. Mazza JE, Newman MJ, Sims TN: Clinical and antimicrobial effect of stannous fluoride on periodontitis. *J Clin Periodontol,* 8:203–212, 1981.
12. Bodey GP, Freireich EJ Frei E III: Studies of patients in a laminar air flow unit. *Cancer* 24:972–980, 1969.
13. Bruya MA, Madeira NP: Stomatitis after chemotherapy. *Nursing* 75:1349–1351, 1975.
14. Sonis ST, Sonis A, Lieberman A: Oral complications in patients receiving treatment for malignancies other than of the head and neck. *J Am Dent Assoc* 97:468–472, 1978.
15. Laforce FM, et al.: Human oral defenses against gram-negative rods. Am Rev Respir Dis 114:929–935, 1976.
16. Shannon IL, Trodahl JN, Starcke EN: Remineralization of enamel by a saliva substitute designed for use by irradiated patients. Cancer 41:1746–1750, 1978.
17. Angell M: The quality of mercy. N Engl J Med 306:98–99, 1982.
18. Sonis A, Sonis S: Oral complications of cancer chemotherapy in pediatric patients. J Pedodont 3:122–128, 1979.
19. Lockhart P, Sonis ST: Alterations in the oral mucosa caused by chemotherapeutic agents: A histologic study. J Dermatol Surg Oncol 7:1019–1025, 1981.
20. Rosenthal S, Kaufman S: Vincristine neurotoxicity. Ann Intern Med 80:733–737, 1974.
21. Smillie AC, Cowman SC: Pulp and periapical involvement in leukemia. New Zealand Dent J 65:32–34, 1969.
22. Guralnick W, Kaban LB, Merrill RG: Temporomandibular—joint afflictions. Engl J Med 299:123–128, 1978.
23. Brown LR, Dreizen S, Bodey GP: Effect of immunosuppression on the human oral flora. In *Comparative Immunology of the Oral Cavity,* Mergenhagen S, Scherp M (eds), DHEW Publication No. 73,438, 1973, p 204–220.
24. Aderhold L, Knohthe H, Frenkel G: The bacteriology of dentogenous pogenic infections. Oral Surg 52:-583–587, 1981.
25. Dreizen S, Bodey GP, Brown LR: Opportunistic gram-negative bacillary infections in leukemia—oral manifestations during myelosuppression. Postgrad Med 55:133–139, 1974.
26. Sickles EA, Greene WH, Wiernik PH: Clinical presentation of infection in granulocytopenic patients. Arch Intern Med 135:715–719, 1975.
27. Dreizen S, McCredie KB, Bodey GP: Unusual mucocutaneous infections in immunosuppressed patients with leukemia. Postgrad Med 66:131–141, 1979.
28. Baumgartner JC, Heggers JP, Harrison JW: The incidence of bacteremias related to endodontic procedures. 1. Nonsurgical endodontics. J Endodont 2:135–140, 1976.
29. Lockhart P: unpublished clinical data.
30. Bodey GP: Oral complications of the myeloproliferative diseases. Postgrad Med 49:115–121, 1971.
31. Bodey GP: Fungal infections complicating acute leukemia. J Chronic Dis 19:667–687, 1966.
32. Taschdjian CL, Kozinn PJ, Toni EF: Opportunistic yeast infections with special reference to candidiasis. Ann NY Acad Sci 174:606–622, 1970.
33. Epstein JB, Pearsall NN, Truelove EL: Oral candidiasis: effects of antifungal therapy upon clinical signs and symptoms, salivary antibody, and mucosal adherence of candida albicans. Oral Surg 51:32–36, 1981.
34. Pizzuto J, et al.: Nystatin prophylaxis in leukemia and lymphoma. N Engl J Med 299:661–662, 1978.
35. Carpentieri U, et al.: Clinical experience in prevention of candidiasis by nystatin in children with acute leukemia. J Pediatr 92, 593–595, 1978.
36. Ewing A: Amphotericin B lozenges in the treatment of oral thrush. *Practitioner* 199:62–67, 1967.
37. Jones JM: Necrotizing candida esophagitis—failure of symptoms and roentgenographic findings to reflect severity. *JAMA* 244, 2190–2191, 1980.

38. Lockhart PB, Sonis ST: Relationship of oral complications to peripheral blood leukocyte and platelet counts in patients receiving cancer chemotherapy. *Oral Surg* 48:21–28, 1979.
39. Mitchell CD, et al.: Acyclovir therapy for mucocutaneous herpes simplex infections in immunocompromised patients. *Lancet* 1:1389–1392, 1981.
40. Saral R, et al.: Acyclovir prophylaxis of herpes-simplex-virus infections. N Engl J Med 305:63–67, 1981.

8. GUIDELINES FOR ORAL HYGIENE, DENTURE CARE, AND NUTRITION IN PATIENTS WITH ORAL COMPLICATIONS

LISA T. WILLIAMS, B.S., R.D.H.
JOYCE L. O'DWYER, R.N., B.S.N.

INTRODUCTION

Recent studies have demonstrated the efficacy of preventive oral care in reducing the morbidity associated with the oral complications of cancer chemotherapy [1–3]. However, many recommendations for this oral care remain empirically and subjectively based. The purpose of this chapter is to discuss the pertinent dental hygiene and nursing issues regarding such care and to make recommendations based on available data for the treatment of patients with oral complications secondary to chemotherapy. It is recognized that some of the modalities are not supported by research and may be controversial.

Nursing, medical, and dental literature each discuss proper oral management from a different viewpoint. Unfortunately, this information has not been shared between disciplines. The focus of the nursing literature has been oral hygiene, palliative care, and the definition and description of common oral problems since the responsibility for the care and management of oral lesions commonly fall upon the nursing staff. Many of the oral hygiene instruments and techniques advocated by some of these articles are adopted from age-old hospital practices (for example, mouthwash and peroxide, Toothettes,[1] lemon-glycerine swabs) [1,4–9]. Effectiveness of these items has been questioned within the nursing literature itself; specifically, use of appropriate instruments and techniques in oral care of the cancer patient has been an area of some controversy [10–14].

There is little if any medical literature specifically addressing the oral complications of cancer chemotherapy. Most references discuss the oral cavity in relation to infectious

[1]Halbrand, Inc., Willoughby, OH 44094.

D.E. Peterson and S.T. Sonis (eds.), ORAL COMPLICATIONS OF CANCER CHEMOTHERAPY, 151-168.

complications and empiric antibiotic therapy [15–19]. Little attention is given to routine assessment of oral condition, problems, palliation, or preventive treatment.

Early dental literature is concerned mostly with describing the oral lesions that occur secondary to the neoplastic process [20–23]. However, recent literature has focused more on the oral/dental complications that are sequelae of antineoplastic therapy. Most of these articles utilize case reports for treatment recommendations [24–30]. Until recently there were no thorough studies on which to base dental treatment, and at times the dental and medical teams have differed sharply in their treatment recommendations. In addition to the problems related to lack of available data, many dentists are not experienced regading the various diseases, treatment regimens, and anticipated side effects encountered in the treatment of cancer patients. Therefore, they may not fully comprehend the scope of the management problem.

ORAL ASSESSMENT

Oral assessment is an essential starting point for any effective management of oral complications [1,5,9,14]. Whether performed by a dentist, oncologist, or nurse, the first step in defining, treating or preventing oral lesions is a systematic inspection of the mouth (figure 8–1). The primary purpose of an oral assessment is to collect data that can be used as a basis for oral care interventions. The optimal schedule for assessment includes an examination upon admission to document the baseline oral status and thereafter twice/week or more frequently as changes occur. A practical approach may be to identify patient populations that are at high risk for oral manifestations of disease or treatment (such as leukemia patients or head and neck cancer patients) and focus on these groups. The findings of the exam should be recorded in the chart as a S.O.A.P. note or by use of a data collection/flow sheet (tables 8–1, 8–2). These flow sheets provide means for assessing the oral status of the patient at admission and during subsequent serial observations. Completion of these sheets may initially appear to require more time on the part of the examiner; however, their use has the advantage of serving as a guide to standardized systematic assessment.

The oral assessment should be completed by those members of the health care team who will be consistently following the patient throughout the course of chemotherapy. Individuals who may be able to perform this type of monitoring include physicians, nurses, dentists, dental hygienists, or even the well-motivated, educated patient. In most circumstances the physicians and/or nurses will have the most patient contact and therefore will be in the best position to provide frequent examinations.

When considering utilizing the nursing or medical staff to implement frequent oral assessments, it is important to remember that oral examination skills are not generally included in their curricula. In-service training programs are one way to equip the staffs with the necessary skills to perform oral assessments. The purpose of the instruction is to familiarize them with the function and appearance of basic oral structures and to develop competence in performing a thorough, systematic oral examination. These objectives can be accomplished through the use of a slide tape program, slide lecture from a qualified dental professional, or a self-instructional learning tool. Given time and availability, a discussion with a dentist or hygienist seems most beneficial because it is more personal, provides opportunities for question and answer sessions, and can be expanded to

Table 8–1. Oral assessment for chemotherapy patients: admitting status

Physical status	Description (normal)	Description (abnormal)
Level of consciousness	Oriented to time, place, and person; responds appropriately	Apathetic; occasionally disoriented; nonresponsive; unconscious
Breath; breathing habits	No odor; nose breather without mechanical assistance	Halitosis (odor); mouth breather; nasal O_2/mask O_2
Nutritional habits, diet	Normal fluid and normal diet	Soft/liquid; restricted or limited fluid intake; nothing by mouth; gastrostomy; nasogastric tube; total parenteral nutrition
Chewing ability	Normal teeth, chewing ability; normal range of opening	Edentulous with dentures (partial or complete); restricted opening
Oral-care ability	Totally responsible for oral care	Performs mouth care with help; total dependence on others
Oral cavity	**Description (normal)**	**Description (abnormal)**
Lips		
Texture	Smooth, soft	Rough; cracked, bleeding
Color	Pink	Pale; red
Moisture	Moist	Inflamed; dry
Mucous membranes (hard and soft palate, labial and buccal mucosa, vestibule, floor of mouth)	Pink Moist	Pale; red dry; excessive petechial or hematoma, ulcers or lesions*
Tongue		
Texture	Moist; papillated	Dry, cracked, bleeding; fissured;
Color	Pink	coated; patches; ulcers or lesions,* inflamed
Secretions	Thin, watery saliva; entire mouth moist	Ropy, viscous saliva; xerostomia (dry mouth)
Gingiva		
Color	Pink; no bleeding	Cyanotic; red, inflamed, bleeding; pale
Texture	Stippled; firm	Edematous.
Architecture	Smooth; no recession; normal interdental papillae	Ulcer or lesions,* recession; swollen papillae; blunted papillae; hypertrophy
Symptoms	Asymptomatic	Tender or painful on palpation; spontaneous pain
Teeth		
Appearance	No fractures; no gross decay	Fractured crowns; gross decay
Oral hygiene	No plaque or food debris	Covered with food debris and plaque
Mobility	None	Some mobility
Symptoms	Asymptomatic	Pain on hot, cold, chewing; spontaneous pain or ache

*Describe location, size and shape, color, and texture.

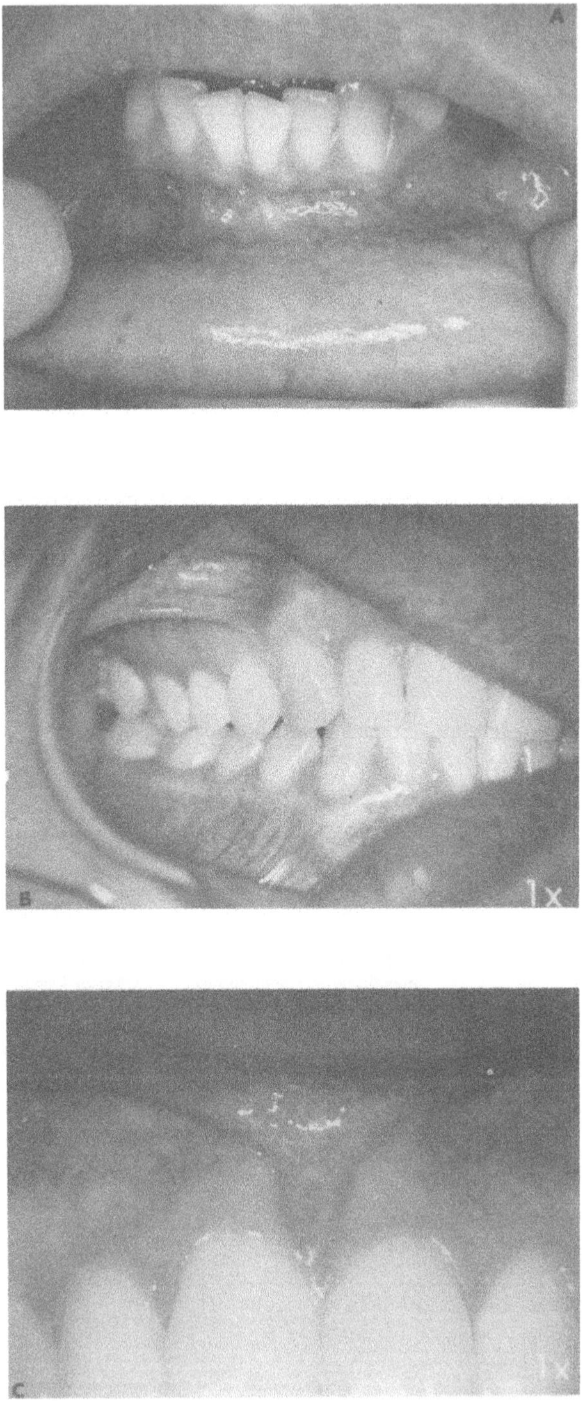
A
B
1x
C
1x

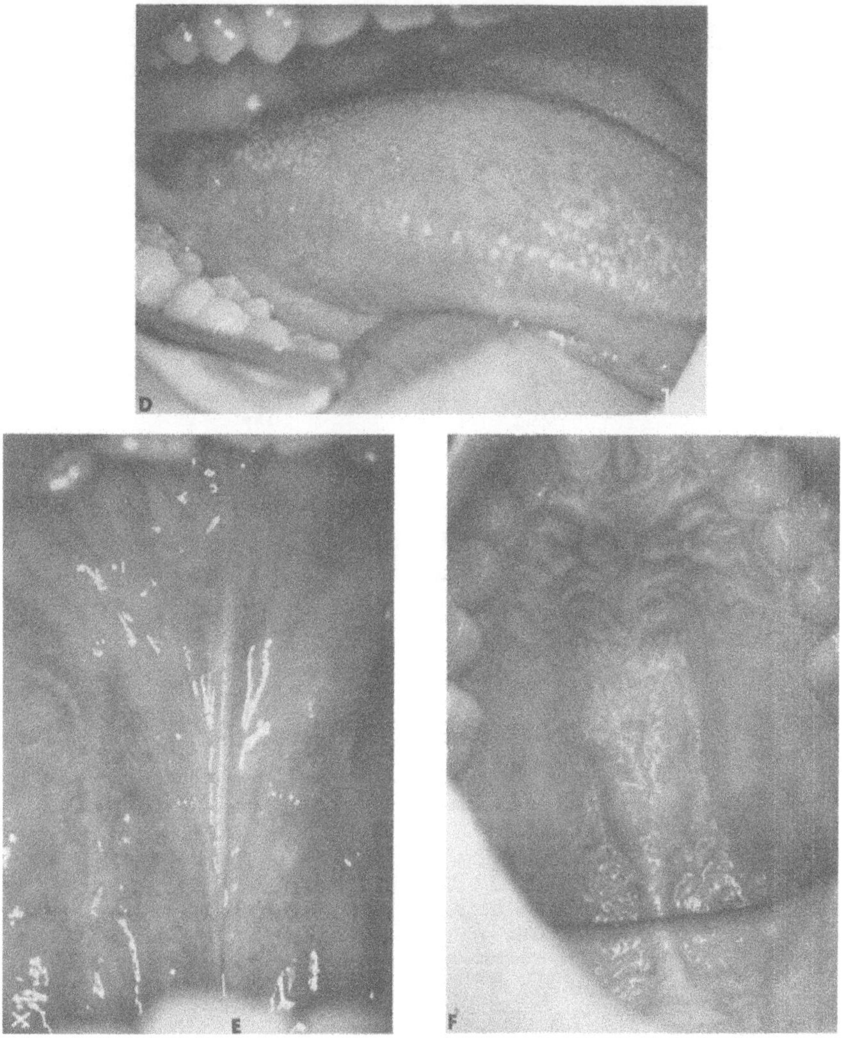

Figure 8–1. Steps of the oral examination.

A. Examination of labial mucosa, vestibule, anterior dentition, and gingiva is accomplished by retracting the lips.

B. Retraction of the cheeks allows examiner to view the buccal mucosa, vestibule, posterior dentition, and gingiva.

C. Evidence of periodontal disease or dental caries may be noted on careful inspection of the dentition and gingiva.

D. Inspection of the dorsum and lateral surfaces of the tongue is accomplished by grasping tip of the tongue, using a 2 × 2 gauze for retraction.

E. Have patient lift tongue to palate to allow examination of the floor of the mouth and lingual frenum.

F. Tilt patient's head back, chin up with mouth open wide to inspect hard palate and lingual aspects of maxillary dentition and gingiva.

(All photographs courtesy of Department of Dental Hygiene, Baltimore College of Dental Surgery, Dental School, University of Maryland at Baltimore.)

Table 8–2. Oral assessment for chemotherapy patients: serial observations

Physical status	Description (normal)	Description (abnormal)
Level of consciousness	Oriented to time, place; responds appropriately	Apathetic; occasionally disoriented; nonresponsive; unconscious
Oral–care ability	Totally responsible for oral care	Feeds self; performs mouth care with help; total dependence on others
Oral cavity	**Description (normal)**	**Description (abnormal)**
Lips		
Texture	Smooth, soft	Rough, cracked, bleeding
Color	Pink	Red, inflamed
Moisture	Moist	Dry
Mucous membranes (hard and soft palate, labial and buccal mucosa, vestibule, floor of the mouth)	Pink; moist	Pale; red; dry; excessive petechiae or hematoma; ulcers or lesions*
Tongue		
Texture	Moist; papillated Pink	Dry, cracked, bleeding; fissured; coated; patches; inflamed; ulcers or lesions*
Color		
Secretions	Thin, watery saliva; entire mouth moist	Ropy, viscous saliva; xerostomia (dry mouth)
Gingiva		
Color	Pink	Cyanotic; pale, inflamed, bleeding;
Texture	Stippled; firm	edematous, boggy
Architecture	Smooth; no recession; normal interdental papillae	Ulcer or lesions;* recession; edematous papillae; blunted papillae;
Symptoms	Asymptomatic	hyperthrophy: tender
Teeth		
Oral hygiene	No visible plaque or food debris	Visible plaque, food debris
Symptoms	Asymptomatic	Pain on hot, cold, or chewing; spontaneous pain or ache

*Describe location, size and shape, color, and texture.

include discussion of basic dental diseases and their impact on the chemotherapy patient.

The increasing work load of the physicians and nurses and the severity of the nursing shortage in most hospitals may continue to prevent the consistent performance of thorough oral examinations. The dental team may therefore be able to fulfill this increasing need for oral assessment and care to the chemotherapy patient. Optimal utilization of dental services requires a consistent referral mechanism to ensure that all patients receive the necessary examination. Hospital-based or consulting dentists who are familiar with cancer treatment regimens and their complications can aid in the prevention and treatment of oral problems. Involvement of the dental team early in the patient's course of treatment may provide the patient with a more complete plan of care. However, this does not imply that the medical and nursing staffs should neglect the practice of routine oral exams but rather suggests that the most comprehensive treatment may be rendered by use of the team approach in which all members are contributing to patient care.

NURSING STANDARDS

A standard is defined as a generally accepted rule, measure, pattern, or model that can be used as a basis. Selected standards are relevant and appropriate to a particular situation. After a standard is selected the nurse can compare the patient with the standard to devise a plan of care. Specific purposes of nursing care standards are:

1. to provide quick, easy access to needed information for nurses caring for the high-risk patient.
2. to meet the patient's right for accurate and consistent care.
3. to ensure that systematic and organized plans of care are utilized.
4. to standardize a high level of nursing care.

Oral standards can be useful to many of those who treat cancer patients. For example, the primary nurse can use the standards in guiding him/her in preparing care plans. In addition, the administrator may find them of great value for the assessment and concurrent auditing of the quality of nursing care delivery; the dental and medical oncologists should find the standards a useful resource for patient care. Nursing standards are not intended to be rigid guidelines for the management of the patient; the guidelines can be adapted in accordance with each patients unique response to his/her treatment.

A format for the nursing standards has been adopted for use at our center from the nursing literature and protocols currently in use at some other cancer centers (table 8–3); [5,9,14]. This approach permits objective evaluation of the oral mucosa, mucositis, pain, plaque levels, periodontal infection, and xerostomia, as well as recommendations for denture hygiene and lip care. The specific interventions listed have been derived from prospective controlled studies as well as empiric and subjectively-based regimens. For example, the use of oral hygiene (brushing and flossing; figure 8–2) and denture hygiene is based on ongoing controlled studies [2,31–35]. In our protocol, Gly-Oxide[2] (10% carbamide peroxide) is used only for the cleansing of periodontal lesions or other small ulcerated areas [36], since prolonged use of a peroxide rinse in similar regimens may cause microbial imbalance. Mechanical cleansing procedures are generally more effective in removing plaque and debris (figure 8–3 and 8–4).

In deciding on a pain-management regimen, we use patient preference as the deciding factor. Therefore, it is difficult to provide data to support the efficacy of any specific regimen. Combined use of topical and systemic agents, such as Xylocaine[3] or Tessalon perles[4] plus codeine or oxycodone/acetaminophen seems to be more effective for control of moderate to severe pain. Not only is patient comfort improved by these measures, but oral hygiene can be more readily accomplished.

[2]Marion Laboratories, Inc., Kansas City, MO 64137.
[3]Astra, Worcester, MA, 01606.
[4]R.P. Scherer Laboratories, Detroit, MI 48213.

Table 8–3. Standards for oral care

Instructions
1. Assessed hospitalized patient will have a documented plan for oral care. The care plan will integrate interventions based upon oral assessment. 2. Oral care is performed by the patient. The nurse is responsible for assisting or completing oral care dependent on patient status. 3. The oral status is initially assessed and charted on the oral assessment data base sheet. The patients that are to be assessed include: a. Newly diagnosed leukemics b. Head and neck carcinoma patients c. Granulocytopenic and febrile patients with undocumented sources of infection (fevers of unknown origin). d. Those being treated with a protocol known to produce gastrointestinal toxicities. 4. Oral status is assessed biweekly during hospitalization. The status of the assessment is to be documented in the progress note whether or not a change has occurred.

Assessment	Nursing intervention
Normal mucosa	
Oral mucosa is pink, moist; absent of lesions, crusts, or hard debris	Mouthwash before and after meals and as needed. To be located at bedside NaCl 0.9% (1 tsp NaCl to 16 oz H_2O) Cepacol[a] diluted with water in 1:5 ratio
Mucositis	
Oral mucosa is red, shiny, edematous, has tendency to bleed, open areas, oral ulcerations. Tongue is red, dry, swollen; white-brownish coating present	Oral ulcerations on initial presentations to the mouth must be cultured. Rinse mouth with normal saline every two to four hours while awake and at least every six hours during sleeping hours. Betadine mouthwash can be used in place of or to alternate with normal saline. If thick mucus is present use sodium bicarbonate mouthwash (½ tsp to 16 oz H_2O or NaCl). 30–60 cc (enough to thoroughly rinse mouth) every four hours while awake and every six hours during sleeping hours If hardened debris use hydrogen peroxide rinse (H_2O_2 3% 30 cc in 16 oz of H_2O or NaCl—1:4 ratio). Use approximately 30–60 cc (enough to thoroughly rinse mouth) every four hours while awake and every six hours during sleeping hours.
Pain	
Patient hesitates to eat because of pain with chewing and swallowing due to mucosal damage.	Bland diet; avoid acidic and fried foods; avoid temperature extremes. Administer local anesthetic as ordered. (For example, Viscous Xylocaine; Kaopectate[b] and Benadryl.[c])
Pain associated with talking	Obtain order for systemic pain medication.

This approach to oral care has been structured around the concept of assessment, recognition of etiology and delivering the appropriate interventions. Consistent use of these guidelines is designed to improve the supportive oral care of the patient receiving chemotherapy.

Debris and plaque removal	
Natural teeth, contraindications: Gums continue to bleed one hour after brushing. Platelet support problem. Abnormal coagulation studies.	Brush teeth with a small soft nylon brush after eating and as needed. Floss teeth with unwaxed dental floss every 24 hours.
Natural teeth, unable to tolerate brushing due to pain	Cleanse mouth with normal saline to remove loose debris. Floss teeth with unwaxed floss every 24 hours if tolerated. Cleanse teeth gently with a moistened 4×4 wrapped around a finger.
Acute periodontal infection, confirmed by dentist	Brush and floss after meals and as needed. Viscous Xylocaine as needed as ordered Glyoxide applied to infected areas as ordered Systemic antibiotics as ordered
Removable prosthetic devices.	
Normal mouth	Remove prosthetic devices during oral hygiene procedures. Brush thoroughly with a denture brush. Leave dentures out for eight hours/day. Store in clean water (changed daily); denture cleanser is optional.
Abnormal mouth Granulocytopenic patient Ill-fitted prosthetic devices Mucositis or oral ulcerations or oral infections	Dentures are to be worn as little as possible (for example, only at meals and with visitors). Store dentures in clean H_2O; change daily, denture cleanser optional.
Xerostomia	
Dry mucosa, decreased saliva.	Mucositis mouth care Artificial saliva (Xero-lube[d]) K-Y jelly to lips Push oral fluids, patient condition permitting High-moisture food (for example, watermelon, Jello,[e] and so on). Sugar-free chewing gum
Lip care	
Normal: clean, soft, intact; lips dry, chapped, rough, but clean	Moisten lips with K-Y jelly every two to four hours and as needed.
Lips cracked, ulcerated	Clean carefully every two to four hours with a 4×4 gauze and with normal saline; pat dry; apply K-Y jelly.
Lips are encrusted.	Clean with gauze and diluted solution of bicarbonate or perioxide, pat dry; apply K-Y jelly.

[a]Merrell Dow Pharmaceuticals, Inc., Cincinnati, OH 45215.
[b]Upjohn Co., Kalamazoo, MI 49001.
[c]Parke-Davis, Division of Warner Lambert, Morris Plains, NJ 07950.
[d]Scherer Laboratories Inc., Dallas, TX 75234.
[e]General Foods, Corp., White Plains, NY 10625.

ORAL CARE FOR COMPROMISED PATIENTS

The nurse and dental hygienist may provide thorough oral care by either simply reinforcing hygiene procedures in some patients or on the other hand actually performing the tasks themselves. This latter situation often arises when the patient is unable to use his/her hands,

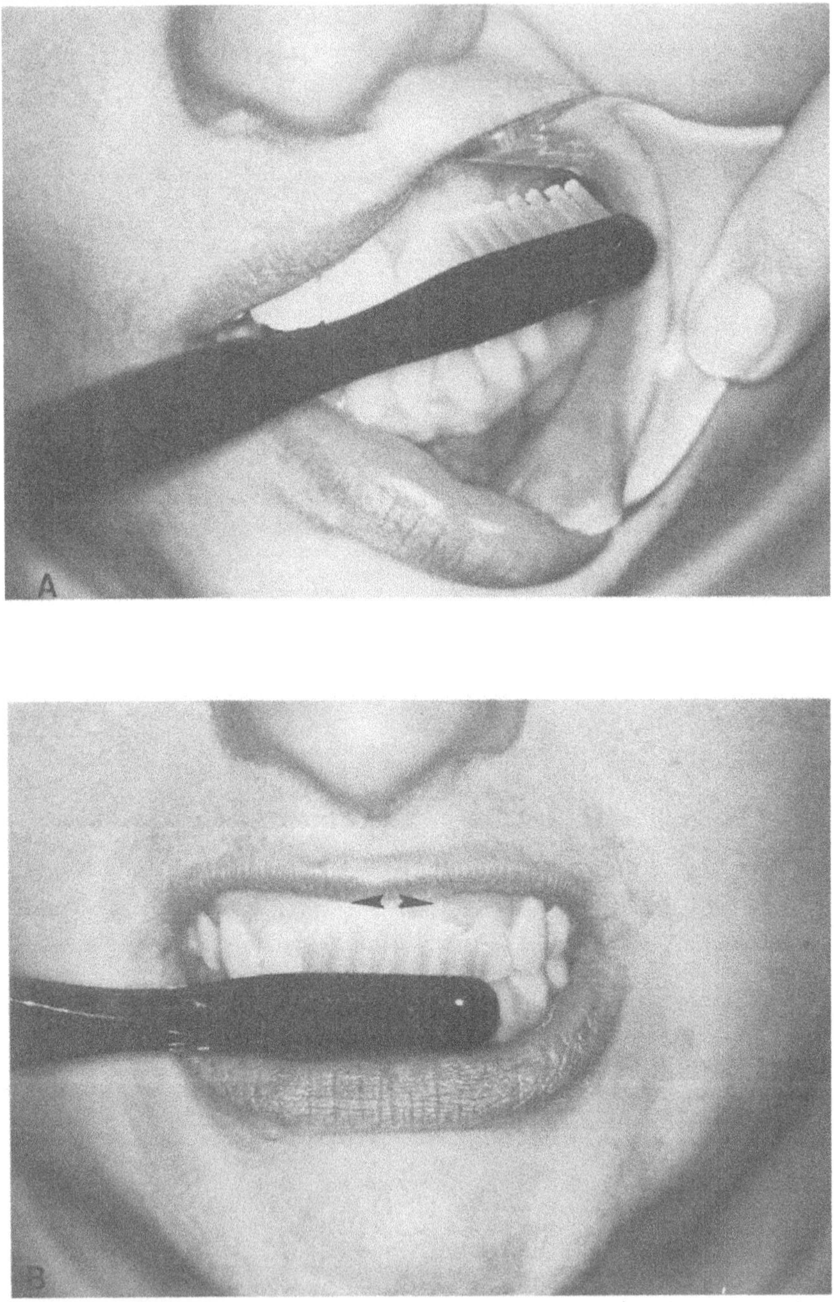

Figure 8–2. Sulcular brushing and flossing technique.

A. Direct soft multitufted nylon bristles toward the dentogingival junction.

B. Cleanse the gingival sulcus area by using small back-and-forth or circular strokes.

C. Correct holding of floss allows use of thumb and forefingers to manipulate floss.

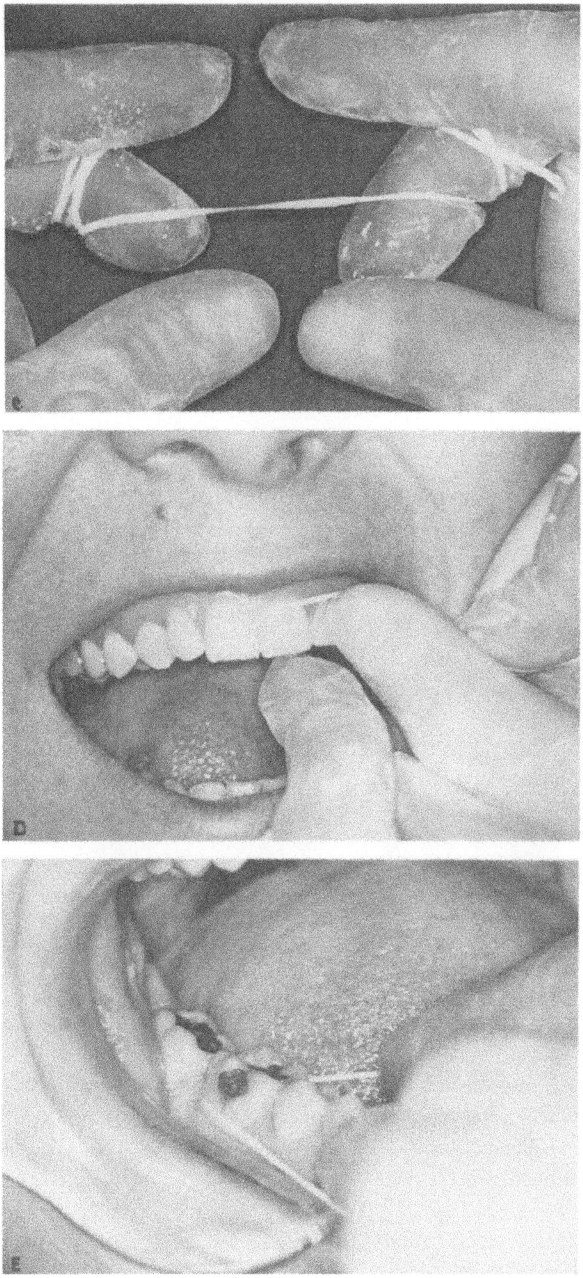

D. Floss is gently inserted interproximally, wrapped around the tooth surface, and moved in short, vertical strokes from the gingival sulcus to the crown.
E. Correct adaptation of floss allows for maximal cleaning of sulcus and tooth surface in molar areas.

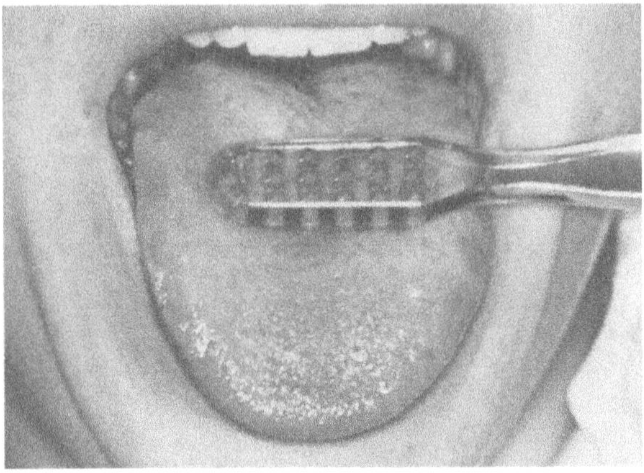

Figure 8–3. Brushing the dorsal surface of the tongue with a soft brush is helpful in removing coating and debris from the tongue.

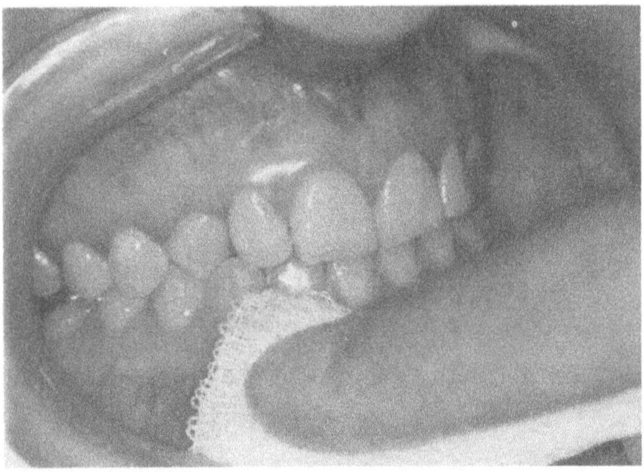

Figure 8–4. Gently swabbing the oral tissues with moist gauze can be an effective method of cleaning an edentulous mouth or a dentulous mouth in which a painful oral condition prohibits brushing and flossing.

is comatose, or is intubated. Although the patient consumes nothing orally, dental plaque will be present [37]. Since mastication normally aids in removing plaque from the teeth, the amount of plaque increases when the patient is unable to chew. The techniques for oral hygiene are outlined next.

Techniques

The following supplies are necessary to perform mouth care:

soft nylon toothbrush
dental floss and holder

toothpaste (optional)
K-Y Jelly[5]
suction equipment
bite block

Oral hygiene can be carried out in patients who are unable to perform activities of daily living in the following fashion:

1. Place the patient in semi-fowlers or sitting position (to keep him/her from aspirating).
2. Place a protective drape over the patient's chest.
3. Position a bite block between the teeth to hold mouth open.
4. Clean the interproximal areas of the teeth using floss with a holder. (Be gentle in flossing in order not to damage the gingiva.)
5. After flossing all teeth, brush teeth; remember to use short, delicate strokes. (This prevents damage to the gingiva.)
6. Wrap a 4×4 gauze around the anterior portion of the tongue and gently pull tongue forward and brush the surface.
7. Keep lips soft and prevent them from cracking by using K-Y Jelly. (Petroleum jelly is contraindicated since it is not water-soluble and can be easily aspirated when used in this group of patients.)
8. Use suction equipment as necessary to keep saliva from accumulating in the patient's mouth.

To carry out oral hygiene care in an intubated patient:

1. Laterally reposition the tube frequently to prevent pressure sores from developing on the lip.
2. Determine that the tube is securely taped before starting oral hygiene care to avoid accidental displacement during these procedures.
3. Follow oral hygiene procedures as with patients who are unable to perform activities of daily living.

RADIATION/SURGERY

The focus of this book and this chapter is the oral complications experienced by the cancer chemotherapy patient. It is important to realize, however, that there are an increasing number of instances where combined modality therapy is employed. Specifically, chemotherapy can be used in combination with surgery or radiation (for example, Hodgkin's disease, head and neck cancer); under these circumstances, oral complications can be severe.

The oral manifestations of radiation and surgery to the head and neck region have been well-documented in the medical and dental literature [38–40]. Specifically, a few of the common oral problems seen with radiation therapy are mucositis, xerostomia, changes in

[5]Johnson and Johnson Products, Inc., New Brunswick, NJ 08903.

taste perception and trismus; however, these may not be manifested to the same degree as in the chemotherapy patient.

As seen with chemotherapy, radiation therapy produces a nonselective destruction of tumor as well as normal cells, often resulting in severe mucositis. Radiation-induced mucositis presents with similar levels of discomfort, infection, and nutritional problems that are seen in chemotherapy-induced mucositis. Nursing intervention is the same regardless of etiology and is outlined in table 8–3.

Although transient xerostomia may be associated with chemotherapy, significant, permanent xerostomia may occur when the salivary glands are included in the radiation portals. The normal serous saliva becomes viscous and ropy with a concomitant decrease in pH buffering capacity and mechanical cleansing ability. This can interfere with proper taste sensation. These changes in the quantity and quality of saliva presumably contribute to the rampant dental caries and rapidly progressing periodontal disease that are common sequelae of oral-facial radiation therapy [38–40].

Aggressive preventive therapy before, during, and after radiation should be used to minimize the occurrence of the just-mentioned sequelae as well as prevention of osteoradionecrosis (radiation-induced osteomyelitis). In this latter case the integrity and healing capacity of the head and neck tissues (especially bone) is adversely affected by radiation-induced changes in the vascularity (for example, fibrosis of blood vessels). Radical neck surgery also can compromise blood and lymphatic supply and, when coupled with radiation, further increases the risk of infection. Dental extractions, deep periodontal pockets, trauma, or ulcerative lesions in the irradiated patient are all pathways for microorganisms to invade compromised tissue, resulting in osteoradionecrosis. This lesion in a patient receiving myelosuppressive chemotherapy can be very difficult to manage.

Trismus (restricted opening of the mouth) caused by radiation damage to muscle fibers can be permanent and debilitating. Nutrition and oral care ability are hampered if exercises are not instituted to prevent or minimize restriction of normal function.

The emotional and physical trauma of undergoing two treatment modalities and experiencing the unpleasant side effects of each can be overwhelming. The patient who is to undergo combined therapy must receive comprehensive education and supportive care from the staff. The critical aspects include initial and routine oral assessment, prompt and consistent referrals for dental, nutritional, and supportive care services, patient education, consistent and thorough follow-up of oral status, and overall emphasis in preventive care [38–40].

NUTRITIONAL NEEDS

Malignant processes may be viewed as having multiple effects on the nutritional status of the patient. One of the effects of treatment of these malignancies with chemotherapeutic agents and/or radiation therapy is stomatitis (as opposed to mucositis). Pain from stomatitis can greatly interfere with the eating patterns of these patients, resulting in weight loss and malnutrition.

The use of analgesics for moderate to severe pain associated with stomatitis, especially if given prior to meals, can facilitate eating [41]. In addition to analgesics, the patient's diet should be adapted to provide adequate calories and fluid intake. The ideal technique is to discover ways and means of persuading the patient to eat a sufficient diet voluntarily. In practice, this is often difficult to accomplish. Increased caloric intake may be accomplished by replacing minimum caloric fluids (tea, coffee, water) with high-caloric and nutritious liquids, such as the commercial liquid nutritional products (for example, Ensure-Plus[5], Sustacal[6], and so on). Some recommended dietary changes to make foods more palatable are listed next. Mouth care should follow each meal and snack.

Eat a bland diet; avoid highly spiced and salted foods.
Avoid rough foods (for example, dry toast). Blenderized food may be more easily swallowed.
Avoid acidic foods that can aggrevate ulcerated or irritated areas.
Have food at room temperature or cool (extremely cold or hot food can cause discomfort).
Supply added calories and nutrients by drinking shakes made with nutritional supplement or ice cream.
Rinse the mouth with a local anesthetic prior to a meal if swallowing is painful.
Chew sugar-free gum or sugar-free hard candy to stimulate saliva if dry mouth is a problem.

If the patient's deteriorating condition results in intolerance to any oral nutrition, alternative methods for providing nutrition are necessary. Patients with functioning gastrointestinal tracts who are unable to orally ingest nutrients sufficient to meet their metabolic needs will benefit from nasogastric or nasoduodenal tube feedings. A preferred tube for feeding is a small-caliber, soft polyurethane catheter (Entriflex[7]). This tube must be maintained until the patient can tolerate liquids in sufficient quantities to meet energy requirements. This form of nutritional support should be monitored as carefully as intravenous nutrition. If tube feeding is either unsuccessful or patient refuses, total parenteral nutrition (TPN) is the next alternative.

TPN is intended for patients having nonfunctional gastrointestinal tracts and is delivered through either a central venous catheter or a Hickman catheter [42] (figure 8–5). The combination therapy of intravenous fat emulsion (Intralipid[8]), high concentrations of dextrose and amino acids, minerals, vitamins, and trace elements make it possible to infuse the necessary calories in minimal of amounts of fluids daily. Administration of TPN must be supervised by trained individuals.

An important consultant in the management of these dietary problems is the nutritionist. This individual is educated to review and assess nutritional status, recommend nutritional therapy, and educate the patient on their total nutritional needs. By utilizing such expertise, the nutritional needs of the patient can be most effectively met.

When discussing malnutrition in the cancer patient, prevention is the key word. As stated by Aker, "the cost of rehabilitating the malnourished cancer patient far exceeds the costs of preventative nutritional support" [43].

[5]Ross Laboratories, Columbus, OH 43216.
[6]Mead Johnson, Evansville, IN 47721.
[7]Biosearch Medical Products Inc., Somerville, NJ 08876.
[8]Cutter Laboratories, Inc., Berkeley, CA 94710.

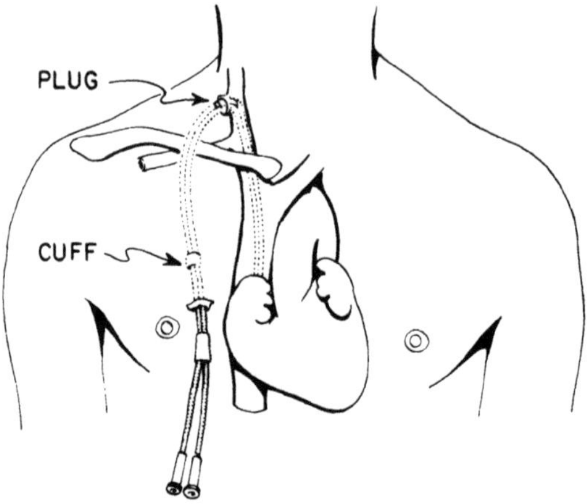

Figure 8–5. Hickman catheter, an alternate method for venous access used frequently in oncology patients, can be used to administer hyperalimentation. (Illustration courtesy Dr. W. P. Reed)

PATIENT EDUCATION IN ORAL CARE PRACTICES

Patient noncompliance with oral care practices is an unresolved therapeutic problem confronting nursing, medical, and dental professionals. One of the causes of noncompliance in patients appears to be lack of knowledge of the importance of oral care.

Patient education involves more than reporting information. The nurse should assist the patient in recognizing, analyzing, and systematically bringing together health information. Compliance with instruction may in turn reduce readmission days [44]. According to Skillern, "the objectives of patient education are: (1) to increase the patient's understanding of his medical condition and (2) to point out his responsibility in maintaining his health and treatment of his illness. In such a program, the informed patient becomes an essential member of the health care team" [45].

The educator must select the method and media that will help patients to reach these objectives. The following is a general description of the method used at our center to obtain the objectives:

Verbal instructions as well as actual demonstrations are used to teach baseline knowledge and motor skills. A well-planned visual demonstration establishes the method in which a skill is done. Accuracy is important when demonstrating if a patient is to learn the correct technique. Time is taken in demonstrating so that the patient will grasp it completely. In demonstrating, care is taken to ensure that the patient is in a position that they can hear and see clearly.

Practice is the next stage after demonstration. Enough practice time should be given so that the patient is able to perform the procedure correctly. Evaluations at appropriate intervals should be used to reinforce the learning of the correct skills since "patients with chronic illness need periodic reteaching" [46].

Oral-care pamphlets designed for patients can be used to reinforce the verbal teaching completed by the nurse and the dental hygienist. These educational pamphlets must be designed around sound educational principles. Verbal instructions and reinforcement for following instructions in the pamphlet are necessary. Explicit messages and correct reinforcement need to be combined with consideration of the environmental factors that can help or hinder the patient in effecting the behavior change [47].

SUMMARY

This chapter has summarized the basic concepts of nursing and hygiene care from preventive, palliative, and therapeutic aspects. Although in recent years progress has been made regarding the recognition and management of oral problems of the chemotherapy patient, continued improvement is needed. The use of standardized oral assessment and nursing care instructions will enhance the oral care of these patients.

Further controlled clinical trials are needed as well. Future areas for prospective studies include nutrition and its relationship to the oral status and the development of techniques to inhibit the development of chemotherapy-induced mucositis.

REFERENCES

1. Beck S: Impact of a systematic oral care protocol on stomatitis after chemotherapy. Cancer Nurs 2:185–199, 1979.
2. Overholser CD, Peterson DE, Williams LT, Schimpff SC: Periodontal infection in patients with acute nonlymphocytic leukemia: prevalence of acute exacerbations. Arch Intern Med 142:551–554, 1982.
3. Hickey AJ, Toth BB, Lindquist SB: Effect of intravenous hyperalimentation and oral care on the development of oral stomatitis during cancer chemotherapy. J Prosthet Dent 47:188–193, 1982.
4. Gullo S: Chemotherapy: what to do about special side effects. Reg Nurse 38:30–32, 1975.
5. Bruya MA, Madeira NP: Stomatitis after chemotherapy. Am J Nurs 75:1349–1352, 1975.
6. Marino EB, LeBlanc DH: Cancer chemotherapy. Nursing 5:22–33, 1975.
7. Daeffler R: Oral hygiene measures for patients with cancer (I). Cancer Nurs 3:347–356, 1980.
8. Lane CG: Nursing management: cancer chemotherapy. J Nurs Care 13:7–11, 1980.
9. Ostchega Y: Preventing and treating cancer chemotherapy's oral complications. Nursing 10:47–52, 1980.
10. Passos JY, Brand LM: Effects of agents used for oral hygiene. Nurse Res 15:196–202, 1966.
11. Van Drimmelen J, Rollins HF: Evaluation of a commonly used oral hygiene agent. Nurse Res 18:327–332, 1969.
12. Harris MD: Tools for mouth care. Nurs Times 76:340–342, 1980.
13. Daeffler R: Oral hygiene measures for patients with cancer (II). Cancer Nurs 4:427–432, 1980.
14. Daeffler R: Oral hygiene measures for patients with cancer (III). Cancer Nurs 4:29–35, 1981.
15. Williams C, Whitehouse JMA, Lister TA, Wrigley PFM: Oral anticandidal prophylaxis in patients undergoing chemotherapy for acute leukemia. Med Ped Oncol 3:275–280, 1977.
16. Carpenturi U, Haggard ME, Lockhart LH, Box QT, West EF: Clinical experience in prevention of candidiasis by nystatin in children with acute lymphocytic leukemia. J Pedodont 92:593–595, 1978.
17. Adrian RM, Hood AF, Skarin AT: Mucocutaneous reactions to antineoplastic agents. Cancer J Clin 30:-142–157, 1980.
18. Dreizen S, McCredie KB, Keating MJ: Chemotherapy-induced oral mucositis in adult leukemia. Postgrad Med 69: 103–112, 1981.
19. Izutsu KT, Truelove EL, Bleyer WA, Anderson WM, Schubert MM, Rice JC: Whole saliva albumin as an indicator of stomatitis in cancer therapy patients. Cancer 48: 1450–1454, 1981.
20. Bhaskar SN: *Synopsis of Oral Pathology,* 4th ed, St. Louis, C.V. Mosby Co., 1973, p 482.
21. Kerr DA, Ash M, Millard D: *Oral Diagnosis,* 4th ed, St. Louis, C.V. Mosby Co., 1974, pp 180–314.
22. Sela MN, Pisanti S: Early diagnosis and treatment of patients with leukemia: a dental problem. J Oral Med 32:46–50, 1977.
23. Deasy MJ, Vogel RI, Annes IK, Simon BI: Periodontal disease associated with preleukemic syndrome. J Periodont 47:41–45, 1976.
24. Segelman AE, Doku HC: Treatment of the oral complications of leukemia. J Oral Surg 35:469–477, 1977.

25. Dreizen S: Stomatotoxic manifestations of cancer chemotherapy. J Prosthet Dent 40:650–655, 1978.
26. Sonis ST, Sonis AL, Lieberman A: Oral complications in patients receiving treatment for malignancies other than of the head and neck. J Am Dent Assoc 97:468–472, 1978.
27. Goepfert H, Toth BB: Head and neck complications of systemic cancer chemotherapy. Laryngoscope 89: 315–319, 1979.
28. Krutchick AN, Tashima CK, Hortobagyi GN: Periodontal disease: predisposing factor to chemotherapy-induced stomatitis. South Med J 72:1020–1021, 1979.
29. Lockhart PB, Sonis ST: Relationship of oral complications to peripheral blood leukocyte and platelet counts in patients receiving cancer chemotherapy. Oral Surg 48:21–28, 1979.
30. Sonis A, Sonis S: Oral complications of cancer chemotherapy in pediatric patients. J Pedodont 3:122–128, 1979.
31. Peterson DE, Overholser CD, Williams LT, Newman KA, Schimpff SC, Hahn DM, Wiernik PH: Reduced infections in patients with acute nonlymphocytic leukemia following rigorous oral hygiene. Proc Am Soc Clin Oncol 21:438, 1980.
32. DePaola LG, Minah GE: Isolation of pathogenic microorganisms on dentures of immunosuppressed cancer patients. Proc J Dent Res 60:328, 1981.
33. DePaola LG, Minah GE, Young VM: Evaluation of denture disinfectants for immunosuppressed patients. Proc Am Soc Micro 1981.
34. Peterson DE, Overholser CD, Schimpff SC, Williams LT, Newman KA: Relationship of intensive oral hygiene to systemic complications in acute leukemia patients. Proc Am Fed Clin Res 29:440A, 1981.
35. DePaola LG, Minah GE: Growth of potential pathogens in denture soaking fluid of myelosuppressed cancer patients. Proc J Dent Res 61:311, 1982.
36. Wennstrom J, Lindhe J: Effect of hydrogen peroxide on developing plaque and gingivitis in man. J Clin Periodontol 6:115–130, 1979.
37. Wilkens EM: *Clinical Practice of the Dental Hygienist* 4th ed., Philadelphia, Lea & Febiger, 1976, pp 242–243.
38. Carl W, Schaaf NG: Dental care for the cancer patient. J Surg Oncol 6:293–309, 1974.
39. Carl W: Dental management of head and neck cancer patients. J Surg Oncol 15:265–281, 1980.
40. Carl W: Dental management and prosthetic rehabilitation of patients with head and neck cancer patients. Head Neck Surg 28–39, 1980.
41. DeWys WD, Herbst SH: Oral feedings in the nutritional management of the cancer patient. Cancer Res 37:2429–2431, 1977.
42. Wade JC, Newman KA, Schimpff SC, et al.: Two methods for improved venous access in acute leukemia patients. JAMA 246:140–144, 1981.
43. Aker SN: Oral feedings in the cancer patient. Cancer 43:2103–2107, 1979.
44. Rosenberg SG: A case for patient education. Hosp Formul Manag 6:14–17, 1971.
45. Skillern PG: A planned system of patient education. JAMA 238:878–879, 1977.
46. Redman B: Curriculum in patient education. Am J Nurs 78:1363–1366, 1978.
47. Still RP, Trinca CE: Effect of audiovisual and written instruction on drug knowledge, understanding and compliance. Pharm Manag 151:134–142, 1979.

9. ESTABLISHMENT OF A COMPREHENSIVE ORAL ONCOLOGY PROGRAM: SERVICES, FACILITIES, AND MANAGEMENT

C. DANIEL OVERHOLSER, JR, D.D.S., M.S.D.

INTRODUCTION

The impact of oral disease on the course and survival of the chemotherapy patient is becoming increasingly recognized. Before such acceptance became widespread, the role of dentistry in oncology was chiefly confined to the management of patients with head and neck cancer; such treatment consisted primarily of extractions prior to radiation therapy and prosthetic rehabilitation postoperatively. The expanded use of chemotherapy in the treatment of neoplasia has greatly increased the need for the dental evaluation and treatment of these patients at all stages of such treatment. While definition of this need has been recently established by numerous articles, the most appropriate dental management of these patients is only recently being described. As discussed throughout this book, this oral management is presently being performed by physicians, nurses, and dentists. The purpose of this chapter is to discuss the logistical and financial issues involving delivery of such oral care services.

GOALS AND OBJECTIVES

The overall goal of an oral oncology program should be to provide the cancer patient with an asymptomatic, noninfected, functioning oral cavity. The difficulty in achieving this goal will vary from patient to patient depending on the type of tumor, its location and treatment, and patient access to dental care. For example, patients with nonhead and neck solid tumors who will be treated by surgery and/or radiation therapy not involving the oral structures do not usually require alterations in dental treatment planning. Thus these

D.E. Peterson and S.T. Sonis (eds.), ORAL COMPLICATIONS OF CANCER CHEMOTHERAPY, 169-178.

patients' dental needs are similar to those of noncancer patients. If, however, the surgery or irradiation involves the oral cavity, a thorough dental evaluation and/or treatment upon admission is important for reasons of prevention and rehabilitation. This evaluation becomes imperative if the patient is going to receive chemotherapy that will result in significant bone marrow suppression, since such suppression can lead to increased risk of infectious complications.

The specific objectives of an oral oncology program are listed next. The degree to which these objectives can be met will be largely determined by available personnel, facilities, and finances. Hooley and co-workers [1] and Poupard [2] have described the methodology needed to establish hospital dental services to meet similar objectives.

1. Identification and training of individuals responsible for an oral oncology program.
2. Evaluation of the oral cavity to predict patients at risk for oral complications.
3. Development of protocols to prevent oral complications by timely treatment.
4. Identification and treatment of oral complications that occur during therapy.
5. Provision of routine dental services to help improve the quality of life in these patients.
6. Coordination of dental care with the local dentist and physician.
7. Provision of continuing education programs for dentists, dental hygienists, physicians, and nurses in the private sector.
8. Provision of in-service programs for physicians and nurses at the cancer treatment center.

SERVICES

Minimal services should include both the pretreatment oral evaluation and the prevention and management of dental complications during chemotherapy (table 9–1). Each patient should be evaluated by trained personnel prior to the initiation of any myelosuppressive chemotherapy. Ideally this should be performed by a trained dentist or dental hygienist, although physicians and nurses who have been specifically trained to recognize oral health and disease might be available. Upon identification of abnormal oral findings in this latter

Table 9–1. Delivery of dental care

Minimal	Personnel required
Consultations	
Pretreatment evaluation	Physician, nurse, dentist, dental hygienist
Prevention	
Elimination of potential complications	Same as above
Emergencies	
Management of complications prior to and during treatment	Dentist/physician
Maximal	**Personnel required**
As above plus	Physician, nurse, dentist, dental specialist, dental hygienist
Comprehensive care including maxillofacial prosthetics	

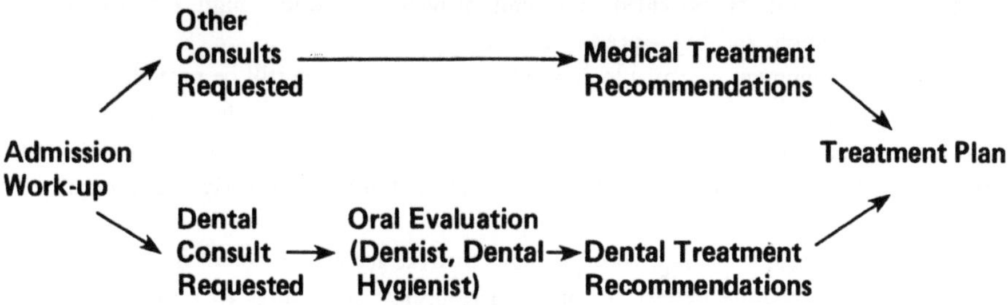

Figure 9–1. Role of dentistry in oncology treatment planning.

case, a dental consultant could then be requested. This type of dental referral might be used in the hospital setting where qualified dentists are not full-time hospital staff members.

Maximal services can be provided through a comprehensive oral oncology program (table 9–1; figure 9–1). Such a program should provide consultations, emergency, preventive, and routine services as described in the following.

Consultations

Dental consultations at admission should be provided for all oncology patients who will receive myelosuppressive chemotherapy [3]. A dental history and clinical examination should be performed at this time. The patient's local dentist should be consulted regarding the patient's previous dental status and radiographs that might be available. Additional radiographs, if necessary, should be ordered. The finding that the patient has no present dentist or history of recent treatment should alert the clinician to potential dental problems. After the oral diagnosis has been established recommendations for dental treatment can then made to the admitting physician, prioritizing the relative urgency and occasionally mutually exclusive types of medical and dental therapy indicated for any given patient.

It is essential that such consults identify problems that potentially may exacerbate later during the cancer therapy. If identified at the outset, appropriate decisions relating to medical and dental therapy may be reached. If, however, such problems are not recognized until after chemotherapy has been initiated, emergency dental treatment may not be advisable or may be contraindicated. At this time, one is often limited as to oral treatment modalities that will be effective. Thus while some dental consultation during chemotherapy can be provided, the emphasis should be on the pretreatment consultation to identify and ideally prevent many oral complications secondary to therapy.

Emergency care

For reasons of patient comfort and reduced morbidity, emergency dental care should be provided as needed for all oncology patients. The ideal setting is in the hospital dental clinic. This, however, is not always possible since many hospitals have no such facility and/or the patient is nonambulatory. In these cases a portable dental unit such as the Porta-cart*, designed for use in such settings, can be used. It can be rolled to bedside where most routine

*Adec Co., Newberg, OR 97132.

dental treatment can be provided. The unit provides air, water, high and low speed handpiece operation, and high-speed evacuation.

If no such equipment is available, limited emergency care can still be provided. Of the range of common dental services often considered as emergencies, the first three categories listed can be accomplished at bedside with headlight and the proper instruments. The last two categories require a dental unit, fixed or portable, in order to properly treat the patient.

1. Periodontal therapy: scaling, root planning to treat acute periodontal infections.
2. Oral surgery: routine extractions and other surgical procedures to remove severely compromised teeth.
3. Oral medicine: treatment of various lesions commonly seen, such as ulcers, fungal infections, mucositis, and stomatitis.
4. Caries control: to minimize risk of pulpal pathosis and infectious sequelae.
5. Endodontic therapy: pulpotomy, pulpectomy, and/or complete endodontic procedures to treat symptomatic pulpal pathosis.

The cornerstone of care remains prevention, however, the means by which emergency situations can generally be avoided.

Preventive care

The benefits of preventive dental services have been discussed throughout this book; these services are assuming an ever-increasing role in the management of oncology patients. For example, appropriate oral hygiene techniques for dentulous patients can be taught by the dental staff and/or nursing staff. Also, after evaluation of prostheses by the dentist, most hygiene care for these appliances can be effectively rendered by the dental hygiene and nursing staff. This staff can also apply fluorides as well as palliative treatments for oral lesions after consultation with the dentist. Additionally, the extraction of teeth to avoid future infection has been shown to be a proper and safe procedure when performed with adequate precautions [4] and is a form of preventive therapy which may be of great benefit to the patient. Most of the previous procedures can be provided at bedside if necessary.

By necessity, some types of preventive care must be performed with access to a portable or stationary dental unit. For example, caries control, a form of treatment by which gross caries is removed and teeth are temporarily restored, should be performed by a dentist to prevent acute pulpal pathosis during chemotherapy. Also, endodontic therapy may be necessary in some patients. Guidelines for such procedures are now developing [5]; with further study, more definitive recommendations based on controlled clinical trials should be available.

Prevention of oral complications of cancer chemotherapy is critical in the proper management of these patients.

Routine care

Routine dental care should be provided at those times when the patient is in optimal health (that is, during periods of disease remission). For example, this normally would begin approximately four to eight weeks following cessation of induction therapy for acute leukemia, when the marrow status has returned to normal. However, some chemotherapeutic protocols include maintenance therapy in which chemotherapeutic agents are given repeatedly over regular time intervals while the patient is in remission. Such maintenance therapy often results in significant myelosuppression, although this suppression is of shorter duration than that seen with induction. Therefore, the dentist must coordinate dental care with the patient's physician, considering any future chemotherapeutic treatment and accompanying side effects. The dental treatment plan must be designed to be accomplished in individual units that correspond to the patient's maintenance therapy regimen. For example, a patient's maintenance regimen may consist of therapy every four weeks. Approximately 3 days after the chemotherapy is initiated, the patient's normal hematologic elements become suppressed, with such suppression usually lasting 10 to 14 days. As these cell levels approach normal (after day 14), routine dental care can be provided for the next two weeks. The dental treatment would then be interrupted when the next maintenance therapy is initiated. Prioritizing of needed dental care becomes essential so that most urgent dental problems are corrected promptly.

Since routine care is mainly provided while the cancer patient is in remission, it can be performed in the dental office or in a dental setting in the hospital. A hospital setting is rarely necessary during routine dental treatment. However, such a setting may be necessary if a dental emergency arises during periods of profound bone marrow suppression associated with the maintenance chemotherapy.

STAFFING

Consultations and emergency care

The number of staff required to provide these dental services for oncology patients receiving chemotherapy will depend on the overall goals and objectives of the individual dental service as well as resources available. At major centers, routine dental care is provided through several delivery systems, including dentists in the private practice sector, the university hospital, and other university facilities. In cases where a cancer center is associated with a dental school, dental faculty will be often interested in providing consultations for these patients. Faculty in departments such as Oral Diagnosis/Oral Medicine, Oral Pathology, and Oral Surgery are most likely to be interested in rendering such services since they commonly provide the didactic and/or clinical instruction concerning these problems to dental students. If these faculty cannot provide such services, referral to other practitioners for the dental care is usually possible. As more and more cancer treatment centers develop dental components, they will become a major educational resource for those cancer facilities without dental affiliations.

In settings without this degree of dental support, dental care may still be available. In recent years the departments of dentistry in many hospitals have developed dental residencies to provide the community with well-trained practitioners with a background in hospital dentistry [6]. These residencies vary from additional training in general dentistry to specialty training such as pedodontics, periodontics, and oral surgery. The attending staff at such programs should be able to provide consultations for the chemotherapy patients. Additionally, dentists who have completed such programs would also be familiar with the care needed for these patients.

In smaller community hospitals where formal dental services are not as common, it may be more difficult to locate interested and trained dental practitioners for consultations. As proper dental treatment modalities evolve for these patients and more dentists are trained in this specialty, this problem will lessen significantly. Presently, those dental practitioners with hospital staff privileges would be the most likely source for consultations and/or emergency treatment. If the referring physician does not personally know of such individuals, the local dental society can be a valuable resource for this information. As noted earlier, dental and medical practitioners in the smaller communities can call on major cancer centers with dental affiliation for advice and support in the care of their patients receiving chemotherapy (table 9–2). Such consultations will often enable the dentist to either provide the patient care themselves or refer these patients to the dental specialists at the center itself.

Preventive and routine care

In order to provide dental services beyond consultation and acute emergencies, additional dental staff are required. Meeting this demand has been approached in several different ways. For example, at one center the scope of dental treatment has included the use of five dental hygiene faculty members working with dental consultants. Each hygienist provides one-

Table 9–2. Dental staffs affiliated with cancer treatment facilities in the United States*

Cancer centers with dental affiliation	Location	Dental staff	Phone
University of Maryland Cancer Center	Baltimore Maryland	Oral diagnosis	301-528-7628
Brigham and Women's Hospital	Boston, Massachusetts	Full-time staff and general practice residency	617-732-6570
M.D. Anderson Hospital and Tumor Institute	Houston, Texas	Dental oncology	713-792-6945
Memorial Sloan Kettering Cancer Center	New York, New York	Dental service	212-794-7644
Fred Hutchinson Cancer Research Center	Seattle, Washington	Oral medicine and oral biology	206-292-7385
Roswell Park Memorial Institute	Buffalo, New York	Maxillofacial prosthetics	716-845-5970
University of New Mexico Cancer Research Treatment Center	Albuquerque, New Mexico	Dental oncology	505-277-6272
University of California at Los Angeles	Los Angeles, California	Maxillofacial prosthetics	213-825-6510
University of Colorado	Denver, Colorado	Sands House Oral Cancer Clinic	303-394-5225
University of Pennsylvania	Philadelphia, Pennsylvania	Oral medicine	215-662-3583
Johns Hopkins Hospital	Baltimore, Maryland	General practice residency	301-955-2083
University of California at San Francisco	San Francisco, California	Oral medicine	905-666-2045
University of Virginia School of Medicine	Charlottesville, Virginia	Dentistry	804-924-3307

*This list is not meant to be all-inclusive but is only representative of the geographic distribution of dental resources.

half day per week of clinical coverage at the cancer center so that many of the new admissions receives at least a dental screening exam. Abnormal clinical findings are then reported to the consulting dentists, and arrangements are made for them to examine the patient as soon as possible. The consultants then meet with the attending physicians to determine treatment priorities. In addition to the improved access to dental care, research data has been generated which has resulted in the expansion of the dental program. Thus advantages of this system include improved access of patients to dental evaluation, fewer patients receiving induction therapy without prior dental evaluation, minimal financial requirements, and initiation of controlled clinical trials.

More commonly, the routine dental care for these patients is provided either by a hospital-based general practice residency or referral to the private sector when hospitalization is not required. In the absence of full-time dental staff, the nursing staff can be trained to provide many of the preventive services for patients.

FACILITIES AND EQUIPMENT

The type of facilities and equipment will be determined by the services rendered. Consultations can be provided at bedside with the use of a light source and a few basic dental instruments. If necessary, some emergency care can also be provided at bedside with the use of a portable dental unit. Table 9–3 outlines the approximate cost and space requirement necessary to perform emergency, preventive, and routine dental services. Ideally the patient should be transported to a dental operatory within the hospital for such care to obtain better access and visibility of the oral structures. However, moving the patient is often not possible for various reasons, so patient treatment must occur at bedside where lighting and operator comfort are limited.

In order to provide routine care a fully equipped dental service would be required. This is most likely possible through an existing general practice residency, or on an outpatient basis.

FINANCES

Patient costs

The overall cost to the patient for treatment of neoplasia can be staggering. Mechanisms to reimburse patients for dental care require the efforts of physicians, dentists, and often social workers (table 9–4).

Table 9–3. Facilities and equipment requirements

	Approximate cost	Space required	Service required
Hand instruments	\$1,500	Cabinet	—
Mobile dental unit	\$5,000	16 ft^2	Electricity
Handpieces	\$800	Cabinet	
Fixed dental unit	\$2,300	100 ft^2	Electricity, air, H_2O, vacuum
Dental chair	\$4,000		Electricity
Light	\$1,100	Wall mount	Electricity
Radiographic unit	\$4,000	Wall mount	Electricity
Panographic unit	\$15,000	40 ft^2	Electricity

Table 9–4. Resources for the treatment of cancer patients

Type	Comments
Information	
Cancer Information Service	Information for patients and professionals on the disease treatment facilities for emotional and financial support. Available nationally. If not in local phone directory call 1-800-638-6694.
American Cancer Society	Information on local resources for patients and professionals
Leukemia Society of America	Information on local resources for patients and professionals
Financial assistance for patients	
Medical insurance	Reimbursement for medical and some dental costs
Medicare	Reimbursement of some costs for those over 65 years of age
Medicaid	Reimbursement of some costs for disabled individuals
American Cancer Society	Reimbursement of some costs for disabled individuals
Leukemia Society of America	Reimbursement of some costs for leukemia patients
United Order True Sisters, Inc.	Assistance to cancer patients with financial need
Charitable organizations	
American Legion, Veterans of Foreign Wars, Lions Club, Knights of Columbus, Kiwanis Club, and so on	All may be contacted for potential donations of equipment, supplies, and so on.

Medical insurance generally does not cover routine dental services, but usually will provide coverage for infection management, including pulpal pathosis, acute periodontal infections, stomatitis, and mucositis. Additionally, such coverage often includes dental consultations and some diagnostic procedures. When the oral pathology is a direct consequence of the cancer or its treatment, cost of dental care related to this oral disease may also be covered. An example of this situation is payment for periodontal therapy of an acute periodontal exacerbation that developed during chemotherapy-induced profound myelosuppression. However, it should not be assumed that the patient's medical insurance is routinely providing such coverage. If the oral care is described using terminology recognized by insurance companies, the plans may reimburse the patient for such care.

Another possible source of coverage is dental insurance. An estimated 33% of the U.S. population now has such insurance. These plans provide a wide range of protection for the patient [7] and should be reviewed individually to determine extent of benefits. The American Dental Association Council on Dental Care Programs has developed standard forms, a glossary of dental prepayment terms, and a code on dental procedures and nomenclature to provide assistance.

There are numerous other resources for the oral treatment of cancer patients. The hospital's department of social work can be most helpful in determining which groups are likely to be of assistance. Some of these resources are aimed primarily at financially assisting the individual patient, while others are receptive to ideas that would encompass many patients in an ongoing oral oncology program. The American Cancer Society, the Leukemia Society of America, and other organizations may be useful resources for purchasing equipment that will enable these patients to receive better dental treatment.

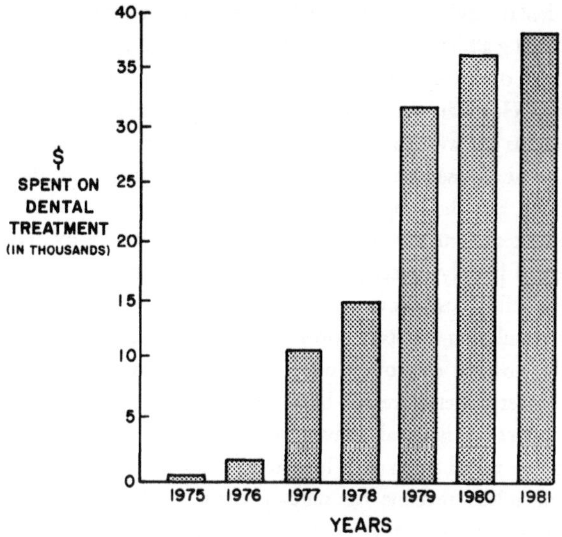

Figure 9–2. Financial growth of dental program at the University of Maryland Cancer Center.

Oral oncology program costs

The costs of such care will depend on the type of services to be provided, the number of patients to be treated, and the facilities and equipment chosen. Figure 9–2 shows the costs associated with providing different types of dental treatment for patients at our center for the period 1975–1981. From 1975 to 1976 dental consultations and oral surgical procedures as requested were the only services provided. Minimal expenditures were associated with this limited care. From 1977–1979 most emergency services for patients about to undergo profound myelosuppression were provided, which increased costs significantly. Preventive services were made available beginning in 1979 with the addition of a full-time dental hygienist to the staff of the cancer center. While costs again rose, patient care also dramatically improved, and many more patients were evaluated and treated. It is generally felt that the quality of care as well as the quality of life of these patients was improved with each increase in support of the oral oncology program. Presently, much of this program is centered on prevention, which, while difficult to measure, appears to be the most cost-effective means by which to provide care.

From a cost standpoint, an efficient program for delivery of dental care to cancer patients is to utilize existing hospital-based dental services. A significant number of hospitals have some form of dental facility. Clearly, any hospital offering residency training in dentistry (*N*-313) or with an accredited dental service (*N*-1,005), should have some facilities available; one can contact the Council on Hospital Dentistry of the American Dental Association for further information. The major cost advantage to the utilization of such facilities and personnel is the lack of start-up and capital expense.

Since dentistry is capital-intense, the establishment of a dental facility within a cancer center may be prohibitive if expected patient utilization is minimal. The type of dental services most urgently needed by the cancer patient is of an emergency nature, although comprehensive dental services are provided at a number of centers. Therefore sharing of dental facilities among affiliated institutions should be maximized. Likewise, personnel costs constitute the major operating expense for dental services; utilization of existing personnel increases efficiency. Hospitals with training programs generally provide a full-complement of services as well as the availability of care on a 24-hour, seven-day-a-week basis.

Funding for hospital-based training programs comes usually from three major sources: patient care, grants, and the hospital operating budget. For most services, income from patient care constitutes the most consistent form of revenue. As already discussed, this source may not be optimal if only cancer patients are treated. Thus the treatment of noncancer patients may help defray costs. For example, it has been shown that more than 80% of the hospital patient population has some form of oral pathosis that requires dental treatment [8]. Additionally, hospital employees offer an already existing population who can use facilities when cancer patients are not being treated.

Both grant support and hospital-derived income may vary. Grant support for oncology programs cannot be relied upon as a long-term source of funding. Such support may, however, provide initial revenue for start-up costs. With the influx of cost caps and restrictions in revenue, hospitals may not place dental operations at the top of their priority lists. As third-party reimbursement formulas have been modified to exclude ambulatory services, hospital-available income may be further diminished. The long-term survival of dental services depends on their ability to be self-supporting.

SUMMARY

Since many oral diseases are infectious, proper oral evaluation and treatment in a patient population about to undergo chemotherapy for neoplastic disease is essential. These problems can be resolved with the help of interested physicians, dentists, dental hygienists, and nurses. As studies in this field develop, recognition and management of these problems will improve. Once the scientific justification for such care has been well established, we can expect that more cancer treatment facilities will be incorporating regular dental care for their patients.

REFERENCES

1. Hooley JR, Zambito RF, Lemmey C: Establishing a hospital dental service. In *Hospital Dental Practice,* Hooley JR, Daun LG (eds), St. Louis, C.V. Mosby, 1980, pp 45–52.
2. Poupard JM: Planning and developing a hospital dental service. J Am Dent Assoc 102 (5):631–633, 1981.
3. Wiernik PH: Acute leukemias of adults. In *Cancer: Principles and Practice of Oncology,* DeVita VT, Hellman S, Rosenberg SA (eds), Philadelphia, J.P. Lippincott, 1982, p 1408.
4. Overholser CD, Peterson DE, Bergman SA: Dental extractions in patients with leukemia. J Oral Surg 40 (5): 296–298, 1982.
5. Peterson DE, Overholser CD, Williams LT: Endodontic therapy in patients receiving myelosuppressive chemotherapy. Proc J Dent Res 61 (March):276, 1982.
6. Council on Dental Education, Council of Dental and Dental Auxillary Education Programs: Guidelines for general practice residency programs in dentistry. Chicago, American Dental Association, 1978.
7. Fact Sheet—Dental Prepayment Plans. Council on Dental Care Programs, Chicago, American Dental Association, 1981.
8. Emery CA: Hospital dental service: a clinical evaluation to determine its justification. J Am Dent Assoc 90(5):1018–1021, 1975.

INDEX

GPSR Compliance
The European Union's (EU) General Product Safety Regulation (GPSR) is a set of rules that requires consumer products to be safe and our obligations to ensure this.

If you have any concerns about our products, you can contact us on

ProductSafety@springernature.com

In case Publisher is established outside the EU, the EU authorized representative is:

Springer Nature Customer Service Center GmbH
Europaplatz 3
69115 Heidelberg, Germany

www.ingramcontent.com/pod-product-compliance
Ingram Content Group UK Ltd.
Pitfield, Milton Keynes, MK11 3LW, UK
UKHW020237160926
475610UK00001B/22
* 9 7 8 1 4 6 1 3 3 9 1 4 4 *